To Be Healed by the Earth

TO BE HEALED BY THE EARTH

Warren
Grossman Ph D

SEVEN STORIES PRESS

NEW YORK • TORONTO • LONDON

SEVEN STORIES PRESS
140 Watts Street
New York, NY 10013
www.sevenstories.com

In Canada:
Hushion House, 36 Northline Road, Toronto, Ontario M4B 3E2, Canada

In the U.K.:
Turnaround Publisher Services Ltd., Unit 3, Olympia Trading Estate,
Coburg Road, Wood Green, London N22 6TZ U.K.

Book design by Blue Heron Studios, Cleveland, Ohio, (216) 397-5793.

Library of Congress Cataloging-in-Publication Data

Grossman, Warren.
     To be healed by the earth / Warren Grossman. — Seven Stories Press
1st ed.
     p. cm.
     ISBN 1-58322-019-4 (cl.)
     1. Nature, Healing power of. 2. Mental healing.
     I. Title.
     R723.G758 1998
     615.8'52—dc21   99-39823
                                                     CIP

Printed in the USA.

9 8 7 6 5 4 3 2 1

Dedicated to Carol DeSanto
who would not tolerate my dying,
but is supremely tolerant about the rest of my behavior

ACKNOWLEDGEMENTS

I am awed at the number of people who helped this book come to life, and dismayed by the incompleteness of my list:

Arlene and Bob Winkler, Barb Israel, Barrett Weinberger, Belleruth Naparstek, Bob Morris, Bruce Cline, Carol Rivchun, Cindy Carty, Cliff Birns, Cydney Weingart, Dad, Deb Smith, Dick Smith, Fran Mayo, Frank Prpic, Gary Golenberg, Gurudev Khalsa, Jane Forman, Jeffrey Bowen, Karen Allgire, Lee Koosed, Loretta Barrett, Lorna Richards, Margaret Lally, Mary Kelsey, Mom, My Students, Rae Smith, Rebecca Hoffman, Rosanna Zavarella, Stan Bellowe, Susan Carver, Suzie Golenberg, The Talisker group, Tom Morgan, Tom Bean, Walter Green.

Contents

Love

The Healer

Healing Exercises   *170*

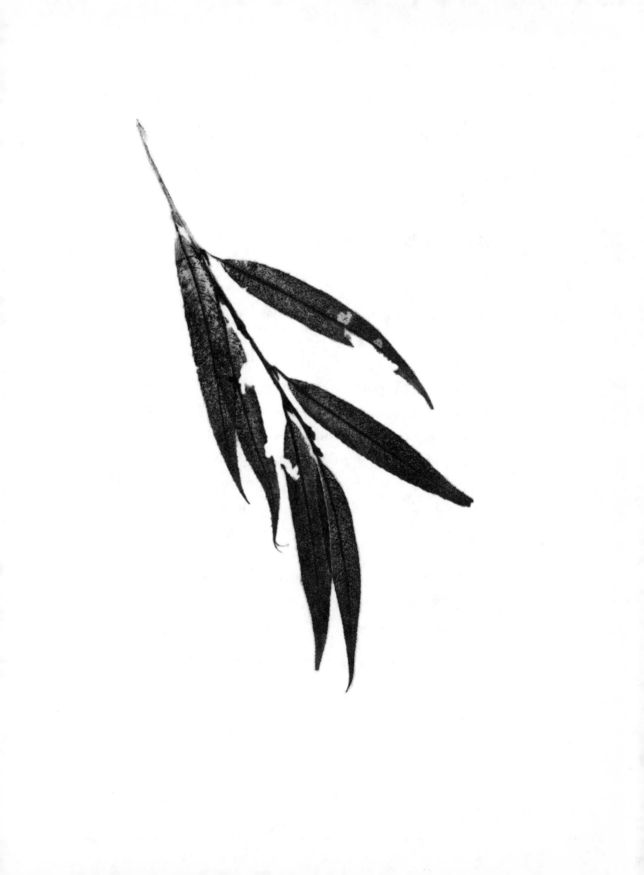

Preface

MY WORK BEFORE THIS DECADE

My life before these last ten years was neither boring nor lacking in purpose, but it certainly was different than it is now.

I started working as a psychologist in 1973. Psychotherapy is helpful to others. My practice was enviable, as my patients were mostly other psychotherapists or people in the arts. Life was good, interesting, meaningful and remunerative. But it is also true that psychotherapy only helps the client a little bit. This is not merely my opinion, it is a summary of the extensive research about the outcome of psychotherapy. Psychotherapy is not a cure; it is a palliative, although a good palliative. It helps people to communicate. It helps them to think about their lives and to express themselves. It teaches them new ways to cope with problems. It does not cure. I accepted this and was glad to do what I could for others in the most creative and interesting way that I could.

I continued at this until the miserably cold Cleveland winter of 1986-1987 had me longing for a vacation in a very warm place. Glancing through travel brochures I saw pictures of Brazil and in a few weeks my wife and I found ourselves in marvelous Rio, surrounded by sub-machine guns, revealing bathing suits, and remarkable cuisine. Somehow I acquired a parasite which laid its eggs in my liver and left me desperately ill. I have little memory of the trip back to Cleveland where my physician said that I had a week or so to live. I chose to go home to die. I did not die, although I stayed dangerously sick for a year.

It is very hard for me to account for large blocks of time during that year. I can remember feeling my energy diminishing daily and calmly thinking, "so this is dying." I can also remember much later, as my energy slowly increased day-by-day. To this day I cannot account for the period of time between those two phases. I truly do not know if it was a moment or a month.

When I was strong enough to get out of bed, it was summertime and beautiful. Each day I would slowly drag myself outdoors and lie on the ground instead of the bed. It was then that my perception began to change. It became apparent to me that the Earth was very much alive; that I lay on an Earthly bed glowing a beautiful shade of blue and flowing with tangible energy. I would stare at the oak trees and I could see their gold energy coursing the length of their trunks. I realized that these huge organisms were as large and as vital as whales. A year after the illness began, I was finally able to walk to the corner of the street. Although I was pitifully weak and terribly haggard, I wanted to engage again in life as it used to be.

Having lost my entire practice in that year of illness, I asked my colleagues if they would refer clients to me. One kind friend sent two of them and I met with both on the same day.

That was the day my life changed forever.

The first client who walked into the office was a man who had been diagnosed as agoraphobic (that means terrified of many things). He sat down in front of me. Utterly shocked, I saw him glow from every pore of his body. He looked like a stained glass window, except for one black spot right in the middle of his diaphragm. I sat there absolutely transfixed by his beauty, as he began to tell me about the unhappiness of his life. I watched the black hole in his diaphragm as it got larger each time he recalled his fears. Suddenly the hour was over. I had completely lost track of time. He left, and my only other patient came in. This man had been diagnosed with an anxiety disorder, a lesser order of continual fear. He sat down, and before we could greet each other, I looked up and saw that he too was glowing. His light was so beautiful, so moving, that I began to cry. Every part of him glowed except for a dark line that followed the margin of his rib cage. Again, by the time I had finished staring at him, the hour was over.

I don't know where the patients began to come from, but one after another they seemed to find me. All of them would sit there and glow. There were similarities to all of their energy patterns, but there were also some noticeable differences. I know that there are other people who see human energy, and many of them attempt to analyze it and heal its imperfections. But I had an advantage. Throughout my career as a psychologist, I had been an excellent diagnostician. Doing skillful diagnosis is like having good musical pitch: it's more of a gift than an acquired skill. I was always sensitive to that slight tilt of the head or that subtle inflection of the voice which cemented the superficial information together to make a configuration that was not merely the diagnosis, but would lead to a plan of treatment.

There I was, Rosetta Stone in hand. At the first meeting with each patient, I would do a standard diagnostic interview on the left side of the chart and on the right side I would draw a picture of the patient's energy. After the first hundred or so clients there were few mysteries left. The patterns of their energies were their diagnosis. For example, depressed people had one of three different energy patterns which correlated with one of three different levels of severity, as well as with the temporal onset of their symptoms. As this process of evolutionary learning continued, I was getting stronger and healthier. The logical next step was clearly to change those errors in my patient's energy patterns—to do healing.

The first way I tried to learn was the way I had been trained to learn anything. I read books and attended workshops and classes. It soon became apparent that this was not the way I could learn healing. Instead, I had to pay careful attention to what was going on right in front of me and do what I spontaneously felt in response. What was being revealed to me was that healing, actually the skill to facilitate another's healing, is inherent in the human body, in human nature, in human intelligence. It is a spontaneous response of the mature and loving heart when faced by a person in need.

If this was so, why wasn't it being done all the time? Why weren't people saying, "Oh, let me take your headache away!" or "Does that hurt? I will put my hand on your injury and make it feel better." I could only hypothesize that in the last few hundred years we had lost touch with our true nature, with our connection to the Earth and with our capacity to love frequently. When the Industrial Revolution began we became entranced with a technological and Cartesian image of ourselves and our possibilities. Now we exist in a time when people barely realize that they live upon the Earth or that they are responsible for its well being.

I earn a living now by telling people, "You live right here on the Earth, Come, I will show you! Feel your feet against the ground"— and their lives change. Now my daily work is opening my heart with love to many people. Their symptoms may disappear and their diseases may even be healed. It was not easy to get to this point, because I had to get past my own acculturation to discover the simple reality in which we all stand and breathe and live and become.

As I found myself getting healthier and stronger, I became aware that there was a definite relationship between my efficacy as a healer and my physical strength. I began and continue to begin each day by lying on the Earth and then exercising, considering it appropriate preparation for my day's work. Healers must draw great amounts of energy from the Earth to supply the heart with a sufficient volume of love to mediate the healing of physical, spiritual or psychological disorders.

Being a healer is like being an artist or a musician. If one has a gift, a formal teacher may be less important than paying attention to one's own experience and to the natural world. Then each successive lesson becomes apparent. This was my experience for several years, until one day I knew that I was wasting my life unless I taught this skill to others.

THE INSTITUTE OF LIGHT

At first I thought that I would create a school which would teach healing to psychotherapists. With experience, the school has eliminated career restrictions for enrollment. We realized that a healer can be any person who wants to be a healer. I gathered together a board of directors, and then I called together fifty of my colleagues and asked them to come and see "a new way of doing our work." On a sunny Saturday morning in my living room jammed with psychologists and social workers, I did one healing after another and finished by saying, "I will teach anyone who wants to learn." Nine people signed up for a two-year course. I was beside myself with excitement.

Soon I learned that teaching healing is much more like teaching dancing or athletics than teaching academics. The healer-to-be must master two skills. One is the skill of connecting to the Earth, learning how to draw great quantities of energy through his or her body. The second skill is learning how to deliberately open the heart at any moment, as it is love, the frequency of the energy of the heart, that mediates healing. Nevertheless, they both occur only within the context of nature, and so the healer must also become intimate with nature. That is the curriculum of the Institute of Light. Students commit themselves to lie on the Earth every morning, to lean against the trees, to examine the herbs and the mosses. In class they learn how to focus their concentration on their feet or their hearts so they begin to develop control over behaviors that do not have names in our society. I'm sure these behaviors have names in other places because I can see my true colleagues when I watch anthropological films on television. All my colleagues who happen to be indigenous people in New Guinea, Australia or South America do precisely the same thing that I do. I have invented nothing at all. I have merely stumbled upon the obvious. I have blundered into an aspect of human potential that Western culture has largely ignored for many years.

As the Institute grew, my best students became staff members. Few people called me any longer for psychotherapy, but many called for healing. I was both amused and aghast. Here I was, a bourgeois scholar in my mid-fifties, and I was a healer. Not only was I a healer, but it was the only thing that made any sense for me to do with my life. I have since devoted myself entirely to this process of teaching people how to love, how to connect themselves to nature and how to consequently be healthier and happier. The Institute has not advertised. The world is full of people longing for healing and they find us easily.

HOW *TO BE HEALED BY THE EARTH* CAME TO BE WRITTEN

I was now awash in this process, with hundreds of students, patients, staff and board members. The simple and obvious truths I had been working with needed to go much farther than Cleveland, as our Earth is in serious trouble. One significant addition to the Earth's well-being is to teach people to act in a healthy, loving and civil manner. To begin the process of reaching a larger audience I started by writing this book. Having not written before, I did not realize it would take forty-five editings over five years, only after which I would then know there were holes in the text that must be filled by images. I realized this in a dream about the book, in which I saw it full of pictures. The very next day I met Mary Kelsey, saw her pictures of trees and plants, and heard about her unique career as an artist in the rain forests of Central America. Looking at Mary's art and at the light glowing from within her, I knew she was the right artist. I explained what I was trying to accomplish and she committed to work with me. This was a delightful six months. Often Mary would ask about a particular topic, "What exactly do you mean by forgiving?" I would ask her to name someone she resented and then walk her through the steps of forgiving. She would then go home, go to sleep and dream. Then she would arise and draw her dream. This went on all summer and well into the fall. By late fall she began to assemble her work and mine into a wonderful and artistic configuration that was superior to my text alone.

NOW WHAT?

At this time I arise at 4:00 A.M. I teach from 6:00 A.M. to 8:00 A.M., after which the students go to their jobs and I begin my physical exercise, as a healer must be healthy and strong. I run every day of the week as well as do the lengthy set of exercises which have become the healer's training that we teach at the Institute. We have assembled a remarkable set of exercises that free people's energy to function as if they were not members of our society, but of some less technological culture where people wear no shoes and live more closely with plants and animals. This is not to say that the students do not go to conventional work places, but they go healthier, happier and more calmly. They know that when they don't feel well they can go to the Earth and get relief and tranquility. As their training progresses they say that their families grow healthier and calmer.

The Institute is over-subscribed. We have a small staff plus numerous graduate students as teaching assistants. We have no endowment and no plan to get one. My healing practice is also over-subscribed. Why are both so successful? The need for healing abounds.

THE BOOK

It was my responsibility to publish this book. We are all in dire straits, as the Earth has been terribly injured by human greed and opportunism. Although the most direct route to aiding our Earth may seem to be through ecological activism, my calling is bringing people's attention to the fact that they really do live on the Earth, that they can connect with the Earth, that they really are capable of love and that they can learn to love with exceptional magnitude.

Who is a Healer?

So who is the healer in this book? Is this someone who formally practices the time-honored art of healing the sick? Maybe, but he or she might do nothing like that.

The healer is a mature person, living in this frequently difficult world of illness, opportunism and harshness. S/he knows that there is a better way, a way that serves both self and other.

The healer is sensitive and responsive to two dimensions of life. The healer is sensitive to nature, interacting with nature attentively and appreciatively. The healer is sensitive to love, understanding that love is evoked by placing full attention in the center of his or her chest. The healer practices that skill daily, just as it is described in the appendix of this book.

The healer is a person who wants to be happy, healthy and loving and works actively towards that goal. The healer knows that the extent to which s/he is healthy and loving is the limit of his or her beneficial effect on others.

The healer may be a sales clerk who knows that opening his or her heart and then handing a package to a customer changes the customer's life at least for a moment, and makes that exchange joyous for both of them.

The healer knows that trivia is not to be merely endured, but is to be experienced as fully as any of life's moments, with an open heart.

The healer knows that there is only one way to solve the truly difficult problems of this world: with love, the energy of the heart, and its permutations—gentleness, kindness, patience, tolerance and ethical behavior.

The healer knows that a better world is possible every single day, but it can be achieved only by assuming the responsibility to be healthy and loving on that particular day—and then by resuming the task again the next morning.

How do you become a healer? Read this book, practice the exercises in the back of the book, and you will be on the path. You might discover that you are a healer in the formal sense, that you have a calling to use your love and vigor to relieve pain and despair. If that is so, you must do healing because it is your nature. If it is not your strongest talent, but you still want to develop it— develop it and heal those in need as well as you can (see the chart in chapter 17).

All of us can be healers, as it is part of our human potential. All of us can assume responsibility for being healthy, loving and good to each other. All of us can create a better world, if we will attend to the two elements that give life and elevate it: nature and love.

Three Comments

1.   Healing is ordinary. In our high–tech culture we imagine that healing is extraordinary, even supernatural. It is absolutely not. Because we are part of a complex industrialized culture, we often lose sight of the ordinary and apparent.

Human beings exist only in the context of nature. We live within an environment and there is no environment other than nature. That environment is the source of health.

A healer does not heal a patient. A healer mediates a healing from nature to the patient. The healer is a middleperson, a go-between. Health, whether physical, psychological or spiritual, is accord with the natural environment.

2.   To write a book about healing is difficult: writing is done from the intellect, whereas healing is not. It is done from the heart. To make this book as useful as possible I have tried to avoid the conventions used in many books about healing. I have not borrowed the vocabulary of any religions, Eastern philosophies, Native American culture or New age belief systems. I have avoided references to past–lives, crystals, affirmations, spirit guides and shamanic practices. The one exception to this is the use of the word chakra, for which I cannot find an English equivalent.

My goal has been to make this a useful guide for healers, those who want to be healers and those who want to be healed.

3.   At the Institute of Light we have found that people can learn to be healers through a process of being reminded of their true nature. This is done by participating in a series of experiences in which the students observe nature's energy and their energy's response to it. They become healers by realizing that they are connected to other life.

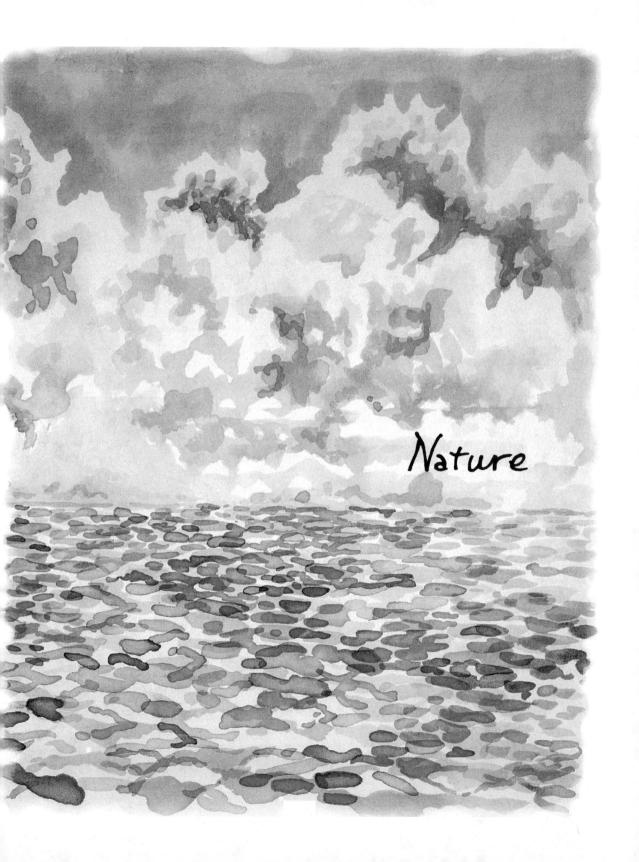
Nature

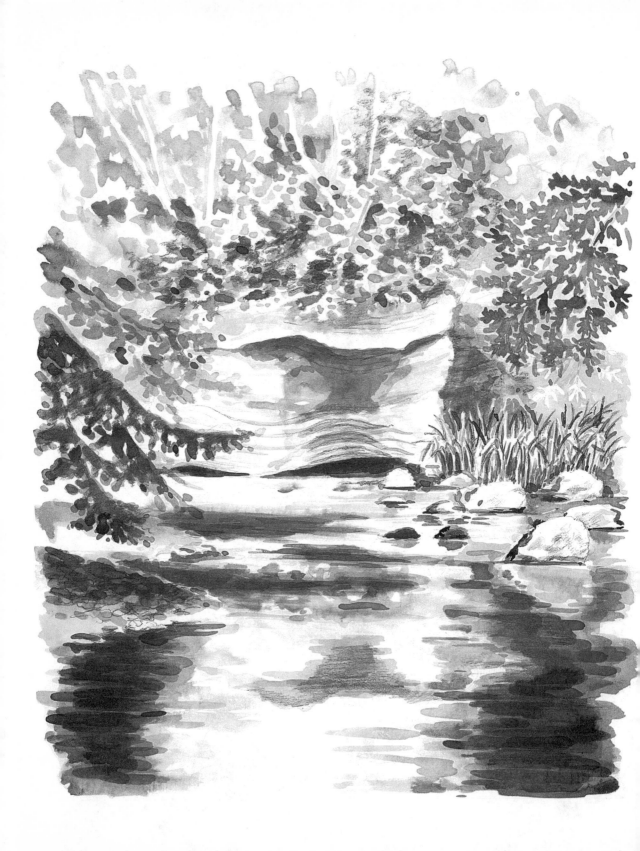

1. Nature's Energy Heals

All people long to be more whole, whether physically, psychologi-
cally or spiritually. To heal is to become more whole. We suffer
from being less than complete. Our incompleteness is felt as pain,
disease, dissatisfaction, anger, illness and fear. We long for
completion.

At all times in history, people have sought healing. In the present
industrial era we have created a technological medicine of surgeries
and synthetic drugs. Although helpful for relieving symptoms,
these solutions do not heal people, as they do not emerge from
treatment more whole than they were previous to the illness.

Psychotherapy also reflects the times. Ignoring the physical and
spiritual, it attempts to heal only the psychological aspect of the

patient, principally by the use of words. Psychotherapy may lessen some symptoms and improve people's ability to communicate, but it does not heal people.

What does heal? It is the energy of nature that heals. We live in and are part of an environment of natural energy that takes various forms, such as earth, air, water and plants. It is from these that healing can come. The healing energy of nature has been recognized by some people since the beginning of time. It has been overlooked as mundane by others. Now it is often held in contempt. Those who believe that the Earth is inert and lifeless disdain their only possible source of healing.

Nature's energy can heal us. This may sound strange if we think of trees or water as matter. However, if we think of them as matter comprised of atoms, then atomic theory can help us to understand healing. The atom is the basic structural unit of all matter; each atom is a constantly moving configuration of subatomic particles. This movement is energy. All matter is thus energy. This includes all man-made and all natural matter and the things that people have created and have not created. However, synthetic energies do not heal. Natural energies can heal.

Throughout time, people have repeatedly discovered the same sources of healing in nature, such as mineral waters, herbs and certain natural settings. Why are these cures not universally embraced? Because they do not work well without one additional factor—attention.

Attention is the connecter or interface between the person in need and the energies of nature. Attention operates like the plug on an electrical appliance; it is one's connection to nature's energy. Without this connection, nature's energies have a limited effect. How does paying attention to a specific element of nature, for example the trunk of a tree, precipitate healing? It induces resonance between the tree and the person. Things or beings resonate sympathetically, they vibrate sympathetically. The person concentrating on the tree begins to unconsciously resonate with the tree's energy, to imitate it. This resonance is the same reason that being with some people makes us feel good and being with others makes us feel bad. To the extent that our energy imitates theirs, our feelings and sensations are like theirs. By choosing the right ingredient of nature and paying attention to it, we will resonate with it. If we do this, our energy changes by imitating healthier energy. It spontaneously mimics the characteristics of the energy of the trees, plants, soil or water. This can result in better health.

This information is too important to accept or reject merely because it is in print. Try it now. Go outdoors and lie down on the ground, placing whatever part of your body that hurts or is tight against the ground. Pay attention to the pressure of that body part against the Earth for a few minutes. Then take a stroll and observe the changes.

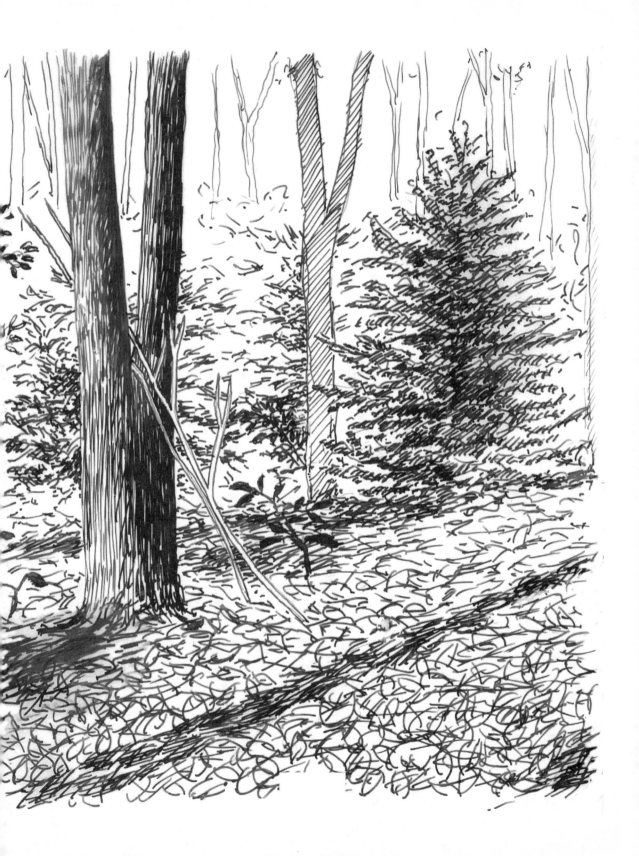

2. The Environment is Energy

The environment is energy. The air around us, the Earth beneath us and everything contained within them is energy. There is nothing but energy.

We are like fish swimming in a sea of energy. We are each tiny energy configurations adrift in a great big energy configuration, the environment. Life cannot exist without a context; human energy exists within the context of nature's energy.

Unlike fish, we have the capacity to pay attention. To fully attend to a specific natural energy is the means to healing (try it; hold some fresh parsley against your heart for one minute while paying attention to the sensation of the parsley resting against your skin; afterwards, see how you feel). When we pay attention to some component of nature, our own energy resonates with that other energy, yielding beneficial results. If we do not pay attention, being in the presence of that other energy yields only minimal results. When something is not correct within us, whether it takes the form of thinking, feeling or bodily functioning, we can normalize that symptom by paying attention to the Earth or plants. In being fully present with that healthier energy, we will be changed by it.

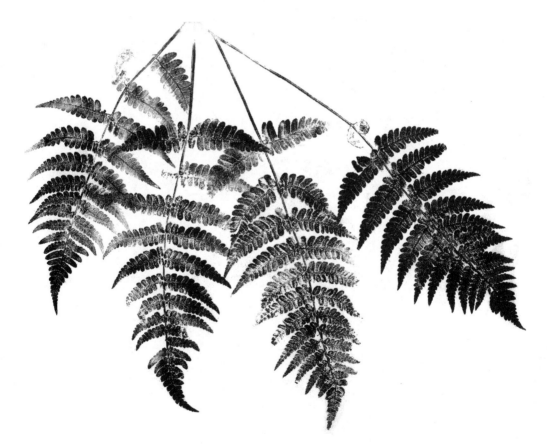

3. Earth

Beneath us there is only one reality, the Earth. It is the principal reality to which the body responds. However, when people are continuously exposed to anything, it fades from their perception. The Earth, being an unvarying experience, is easily lost sight of. It is made even less apparent because modern social and religious practices pay little attention to the Earth, failing to help people focus anew on the prime wonder. Insensate, we take its gifts—animal, mineral and vegetable—and process them or synthesize from them. We then forget that these processed products are derived from the Earth. We imagine that they are solely our inventions, the results of our cleverness.

Likewise, the conventional approach to people in need is to treat them with derivative products: drugs, food supplements and words. While these may be helpful, such secondary approaches are

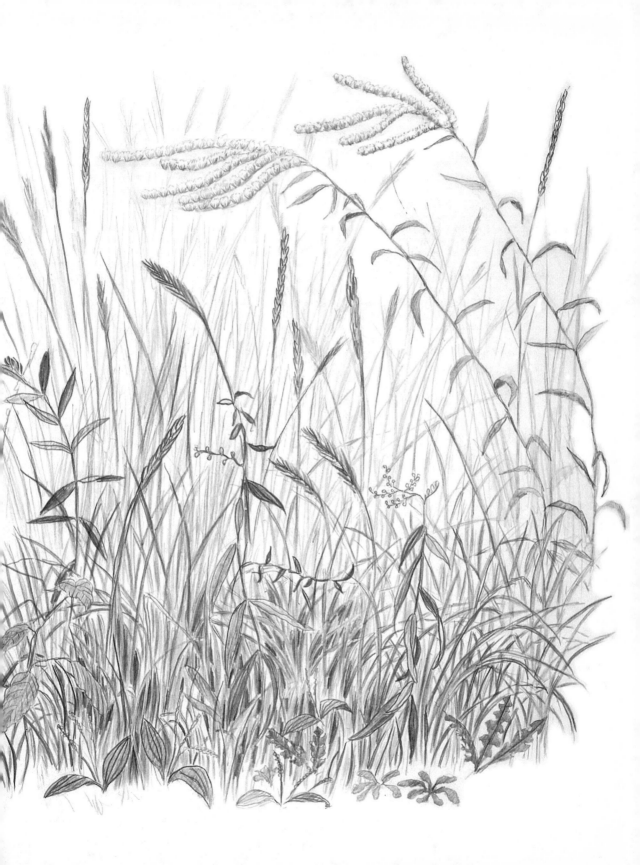

insufficient to produce healing, although they may provide symptom relief. Take heart, we have the greatest of resources available beneath us.

The frequency of the Earth's energy is the most healing of all frequencies. Sit, stand or lie upon the Earth each time you have a headache, indigestion, anxiety or tension. Try the same thing after work each day to calm yourself. Do it after an uncomfortable auto trip. Each time, pay attention to the pressure of the uncomfortable part of your body as it rests against the Earth: feet, back or buttocks. By doing this, your much smaller energy begins to resonate with the Earth's very large energy, imitating its health.

Interacting with the Earth in this way is a significant treatment for psychological symptoms such as anxiety, depression, obsessional thought, compulsive behavior and anger, as well as an antidote to physical symptoms such as headache, backache, indigestion and so forth. Why isn't this common knowledge? Because we were not taught this when we were young. Children bring their pain or unhappiness to their parents. These are the moments in which they learn how to deal with discomfort. These strategies for becoming more comfortable usually endure for a lifetime, whether or not they are effective. If a wise parent would have said, "Oh my, your tummy hurts; let's go outside and lie on the ground for a few moments," the child would have learned a natural and effective solution. One major task of healers is to introduce these uses of the Earth to the patient, who will then bring the learning to others.

The Earth is the ultimate mother. This is not a metaphor. She nurtures and supports us. If a child has sufficient nurturing and support during early developmental phases, s/he grows up happy, confident and calm. Many people are quite the opposite. They have experienced mothering deficits (as well as fathering deficits). In adulthood, the only remedy for lack of sufficient or appropriate early mothering is the Great Mother. Connecting through quiet attention to the feminine energy of the Earth has the potential to reverse psychological and physical dysfunction. Doing this with the added facilitation of a healer or a loving friend greatly increases the likelihood of success.

The daily preparation for all healers is interaction with nature. This is the only way to learn what healthy energy is, and how to access

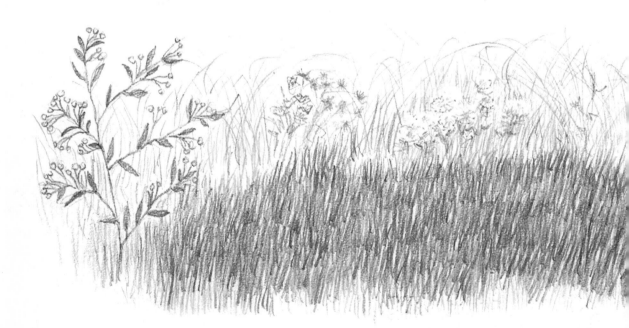

it. An unhealthy healer cannot be. Healers must be models of health, as much of the healing process consists of demonstrating proper energy flow to the patient (actually to the patient's energy). To accomplish this, healers begin each day by going to the Earth— lying, standing, sitting or kneeling on it with great attentiveness.

The Earth provides the conditions for healthy existence.

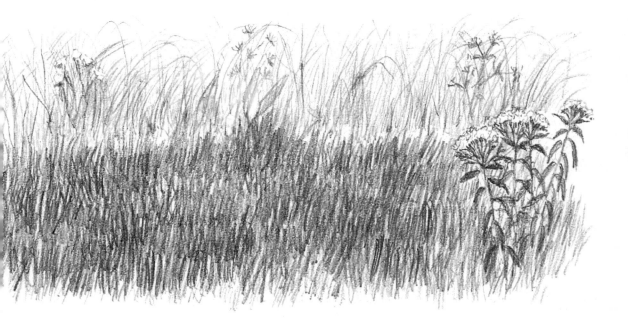

4. Attention

Attention is the principal means for accessing healing from nature. It functions as the interface or connecter between nature's energies and a person's need. By paying complete attention to an aspect of nature, for example the trunk of a willow tree, one becomes spontaneously synchronized with it so a change in one's energy can occur.

For example, in order to pay attention to a tree with the hope of healing one's spine, one might pay attention to the physical sensation of one's spine pressed against the tree. One could use the same tree to relieve arthritic pain by paying attention to the sensation of one's heart touching the tree (the back of the heart chakra is between the shoulder blades).

A healer must be able to pay attention exquisitely. For example, he or she may be with a child who suffers from multiple allergies. Perceiving that the energy of the child's spleen and throat are disordered, the healer must model near-perfect energy flow in those parts of his or her own body. Then s/he must pay attention to his or her own heart so that it expands sufficiently to allow the energy of nature to pass through it and heal the child. If the healer cannot pay attention well, the healing will not occur. One who wishes to heal himself or herself must likewise pay careful attention as he places an appropriate plant or flower against the needy part of the body.

Meditations are structured activities that improve attention. To meditate is to pay attention to only one thing at a time, whether it is a sound, object, image or word. Meditation is not at all mysterious or enigmatic. All spiritual and martial traditions recognize the importance of attention, and each has its own way of teaching meditation. It is especially valuable if one pays attention to a very healthy object. Thus a religious aspirant may pay attention to the name of God. Healers need to pay attention to nature's energies, one at a time. These include different kinds of trees, herbs, soil and so forth. These meditations do several things. They train the healer's energy flow, teach about the world in which he or she lives, and increase attentiveness and calmness.

To pay attention well, one begins by deciding to do so. Of course, one is also pulled in the opposite direction, to not pay attention. There is always this opposing force. This may take the form of irrelevant thoughts, complaints about the task, wishes to be elsewhere or doubts about the value of the experience. This internal opposition to paying attention must not be battled. Anger, criticizing oneself or tightening in control are never helpful. These are "anti–healing" behaviors. One need only pause, kindly acknowledge one's ambivalence and then gently return to the task of paying attention.

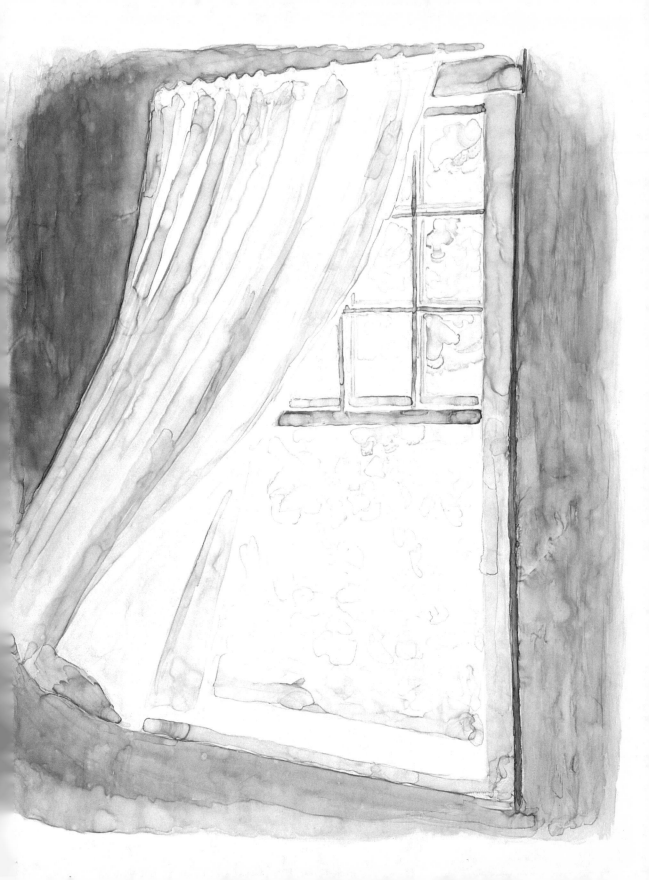

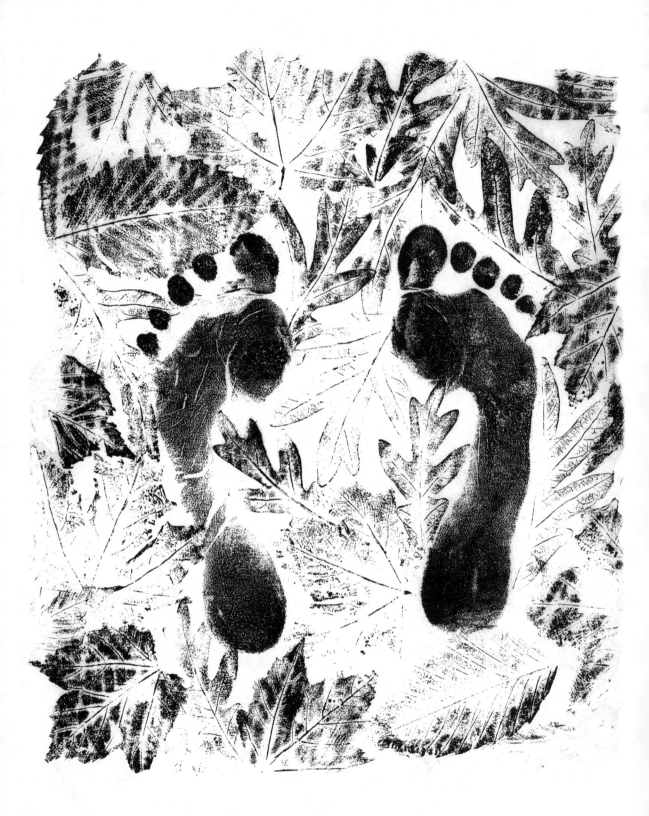

5. Connecting into the Earth

To be calmer and healthier you must learn how to use your attention to connect with the Earth. This will literally fill your body with the Earth's energy. The method for doing this is simple, although mastery of it requires some practice. Stand on the ground, preferably without shoes, while quietly paying attention to the sensation of your feet against the ground. Do this several times each day. In a few weeks you will be quite skilled. Doing this can change your life.

Why should this single meditation cause such desirable results? Because paying attention to the Earth against one's feet spontaneously induces an increase in the flow of energy from the Earth up into one's body. If one practices this daily, one's vigor and comfort will increase as the rate of one's energy flow increases. Even with no further healing at all, there will be symptom reduction and attitude change as a result of a greater volume of energy flow. If one is more energetic, one is less easily disturbed by frustration or discomfort.

After practicing this form of standing on the Earth repeatedly, one learns to do it more efficiently—increasing the energy flow from the Earth into the body. Soon one is ready to apply this to specific life tasks. All tasks can be done more effectively when one has more energy. This practice will have particular significance if one has failed repeatedly at a specific task, such as schoolwork, assertiveness, creativity or sexual behavior. Precede these and any meaningful or difficult tasks with concentrating on your feet against the Earth.

Anxiety, fear and terror are antithetical to this healthy behavior. In all three, the diaphragm contracts upwards and the body's energy pulls up and away from the Earth (make a gasping sound of terror and you will feel this). The antidote to any moment of fear is to quietly attend to the sensation of your feet against the ground or any other surface. This can reinstate the appropriate energy flow and will calm you.

We fill the body with energy by connecting to the Earth.

We heal the body with energy by connecting to the Earth.

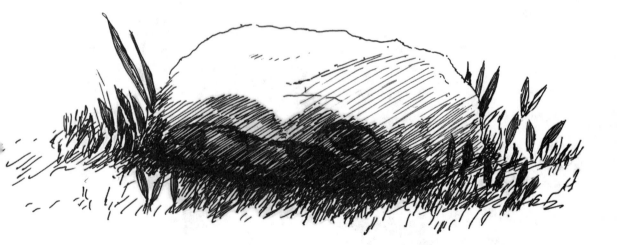

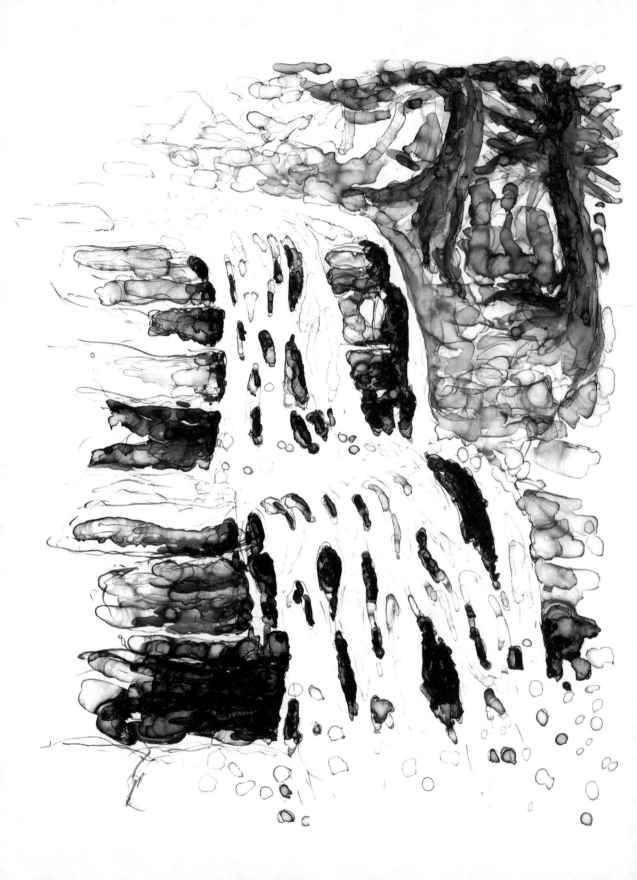

6. Functions of Earth Energy

The Earth's energy performs three principal functions for people.

The first of the Earth's functions is detoxification. People are constantly ingesting unhealthy substances through food, air, water and interaction with other people. The presence of this harmful energy in the body interferes with healthy physical and psychological functioning. What can one do about this? Discharge the unwanted energy into the Earth. The easiest way to do this is to lie on your back on the ground. As you lie paying attention to the Earth against your spine, your energy spontaneously interacts with the Earth's energy and detoxification begins. The spine emits waste energy. The Earth recycles all of our wastes, including waste energy. This general detoxification procedure may not be fully adequate for you each day. Using your own judgment, you may in addition choose to focus your attention at the interface of the ground and one of the following organs: lungs, colon, kidneys or throat. These are areas of frequent inefficiency, discomfort and illness. Describing this process will convince few readers. But the experience of being changed quickly by lying on the Earth is easily available to all who try.

If you use medicine, it would be helpful to pay attention to your liver and kidneys, holding them against the ground each day. If you have a cold or the flu, be certain to do this with your kidneys and lungs (refer to an anatomy book for their locations). If you have pain anywhere, place the painful area against the Earth and pay attention to the sensation of pressure where it touches the ground (this includes lower back pain). Daily maintenance for healers, with or without discomfort, should involve lying mindfully on the Earth first thing in the morning and after work is finished.

The second function of the Earth's energy is filling the body with energy (see the previous chapter). This is an unfamiliar idea in our culture. As one stands upon the Earth, one interacts with it. If one stands mindfully, attending to one's feet against the Earth, one spontaneously induces a pump–like effect in the feet that draws the Earth's energy upwards through the body. Much of what we call physical illness and psychopathology can be lessened or eliminated if a person has more energy. The Earth is the source of this energy. Although we want to fill the body with the Earth's energy, it will not help to try to draw or pull the energy upwards. One can either pay attention to the sensation of the feet against the Earth or aim down through them into the Earth.

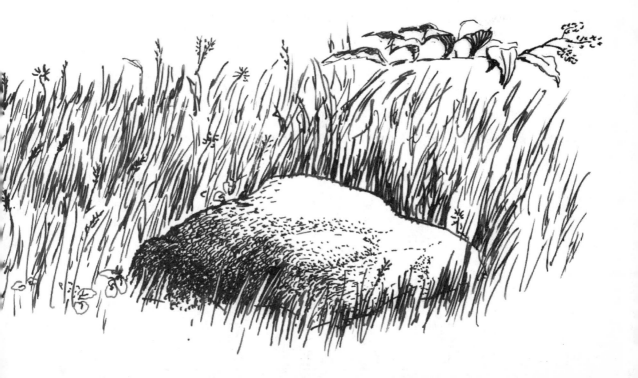

The third function that the Earth's energy performs for us is improving common sense. Many of us spend our days in abstract or cognitive pursuits: conducting business, operating machinery, learning theories or consulting. These activities are unnatural. They are invented activities which engage us in an artificial system of symbols and contingencies that have little to do with the natural use of mind and body. We all have had the discomfort that follows hours of study, writing or preparing a tax return. This physical–psychological discomfort is caused by immersing oneself in artificial activity. If one does this every day, unhealthy and uncomfortable change occurs in one's thoughts, values and perception of reality. Unfortunately, this is the nature of many occupations. The antidote is spending a bit of time on the Earth each day, ideally upon awakening and again after the day's work is finished.

The practices of healing, counseling and medicine are often stressful and consequently unhealthy for the practitioner. The level of stress is proportional to the seriousness of the patients' illnesses.

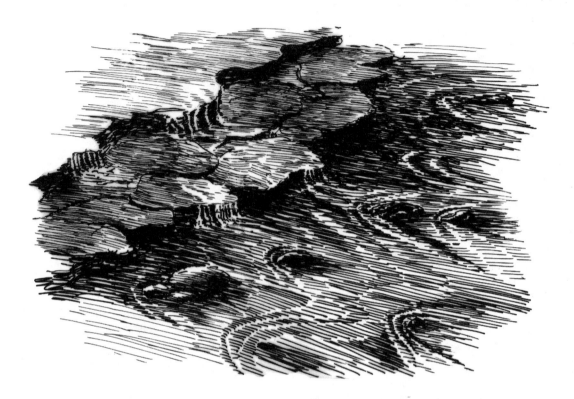

The helping professional, as much as the patient, needs the gifts of
the Earth every day in order to be detoxified and energized and
returned to quiet simplicity.

7. Trees

Trees function as living tubes which draw the Earth's energy upwards and make it available to us in a slightly altered form. Although we live among these cylinders of flowing energy, few of us realize their potential to heal and teach us.

Each species of plant takes the Earth's energy and, in its specific way, makes it accessible for human needs. Trees, with their powerful linear energy flow, can be used to aid us in improving our own linear energy flow, that is, our flow of energy from foot to head. We are also cylindrical organisms through which energy flows. We also reach down into the Earth for sustenance and upwards for inspiration. As trees do this with excellence, we can be their students in a special way.

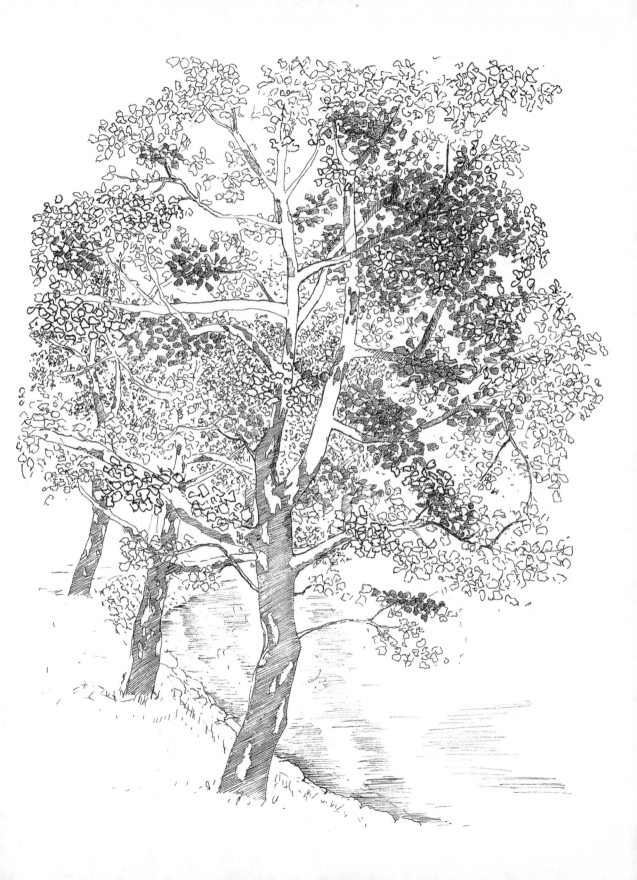

Healthy people, like trees, flow with unimpeded energy. This leaves them feeling confident, supported and able to competently engage in each day's tasks. The experiences of suffering or worrying are caused by interruptions to this direct flow of energy. The experiences of pain or illness are the same.

How can you use a tree as part of your healing? Go to a large deciduous tree and lean a distressed body part against that huge energy flow. Pay attention to the place where you feel your body against the tree. After a while you will become calmer and more energized. You may even have immediate relief from discomfort.

If a person stands near a tree, s/he has stepped into a strong, healthy energy updraft (the tree's energy extends past the trunk) and will be affected beneficially. S/he has found a natural, effective support for his or her own energy. It is also helpful that this gift comes without words or explanations so s/he can sidestep the morass of reasoning.

Each species of tree has a different sort of energy. You will find that the experience and the benefits of leaning against or standing near them varies. Trees with more feminine energy, such as willows or sycamores, seem to relieve pain well. Trees with more masculine energy, such as oaks and beeches, help the alignment of the body with their more powerful upward energy flow.

In addition each tree, like each person, has qualities unlike the rest of its species. With a bit of attention and practice you will find yourself easily discriminating among them, and able to find trees which satisfy a variety of your needs.

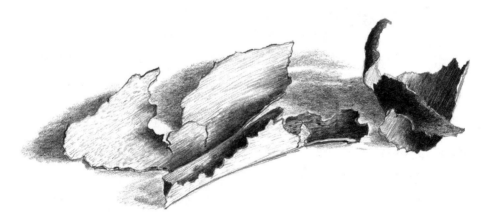

8. Air

Air, nature's energy in gaseous form, flows directly into your body every moment of your life. Your lungs are the delicate interface between outside and inside. It is here that air combines with blood. It is here that the energy of the environment becomes even more personal for a brief time. The wonder of this is repeated from moment to moment all through your life.

As nature's energy enters your body in the form of air, you become one with it. Breathing it while moving through it, you are within a great and weightless healing medium and it is within you. Air delicately cups your entire body surface from the outside while it lifts and buoys the lungs from the inside. In the center of your body is an almost weightless place; the heart rests lightly here, cushioned by the lungs. Healthy lungs provide the emotional experience of buoyancy and hopefulness.

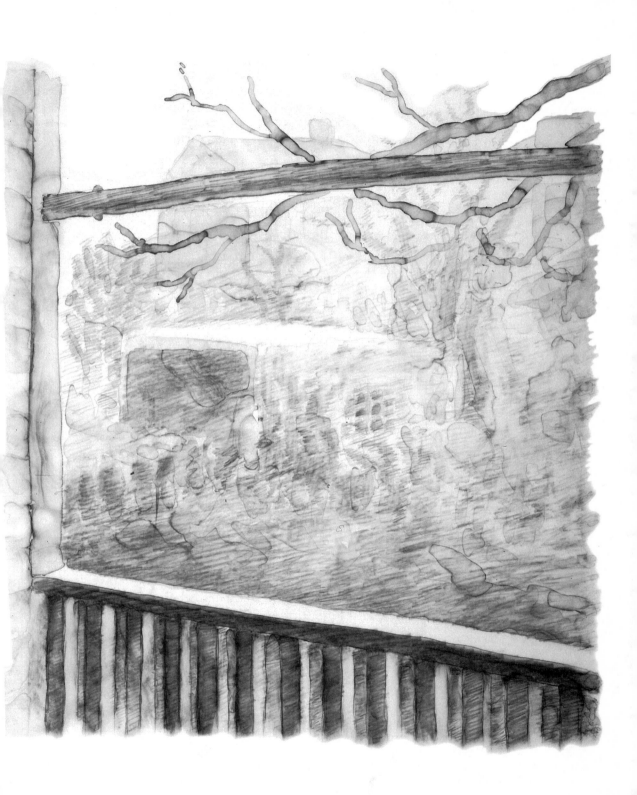

Most of us have less than rhythmic or full breathing. If our breathing were deep and relaxed we would be calm. If we were calm we would have few physical or psychological symptoms. Interestingly, the best way to change uncomfortable breathing is not by learning a new way of breathing, but by accessing more of the energy of the Earth through the feet or seat. This will change the whole body's energy flow, which then alters one's breathing. This can often be accomplished by doing the exercises in the appendix.

Treating a symptom, although it complies with the wish of the patient and the structure of the marketplace, generally fails to result in more than a temporary change. Learning a new way of breathing is a good example of this. It lasts exactly as long as one is paying attention to doing it. A skilled healer looks for the cause of the symptom both within the organization of a person's energy and in the patient's relationship to the energy of the Earth. Anxious or shallow breathing is a physical and emotional state expressed by the diaphragm's limited range of movement. In order to heal the diaphragm, significant healing of the first and third chakras is required, after which the breathing should correct itself.

How does smoking affect healing? The lungs of the smoker have become limited in their capacity to receive oxygen. Insufficient oxygen weakens the entire body, especially the lungs and heart. The smoker comes to any challenge with an impediment to success because the courage to engage in one's life requires an energized heart. People must have enough energy to engage in changing their lives. If their oxygen, and thus their energy supply, is limited, it is difficult to move forward. This must be explained to the smoker while the healer's heart is in an open, loving state. The information has been given to the smoker many times before. It is love, however, that "floats the words" past the smoker's defenses, allowing them to be acknowledged. Then the healer, still with open heart, must clearly direct the smoker to stop.

No healer can smoke, as it takes a strong and healthy body to provide the heart with sufficient energy to produce enough love to help make someone else's life better.

9. Energy Flow is Bipolar

It is only when one accepts that energy forms and controls matter, that one begins to understand healing.

Healing is the rearranging of the energy that is a human being into a more efficient pattern of movement. This is possible with the Earth's gifts. It is made far more likely with the Earth plus the presence of a healer to lovingly mediate the healing, to mediate the energy flow from the Earth.

Although we stand on the Earth and we exist only by her nourishment, the body's energy is bipolar. It flows up and down simultaneously. Our feet relate to the Earth, while our heads reach upwards toward the heavens. The word "heaven" bears connotations of an earlier time and a different notion of the world.

Still, the heavens are as much a part of the natural environment as the Earth. The energy of nature is quite the same whether above us or below. It is human beings whose energy frequency changes from bottom to top, from seat to head, because the chakra system raises that frequency during the upward flow of energy.

What is the significance of this for healing? Healing is the result of

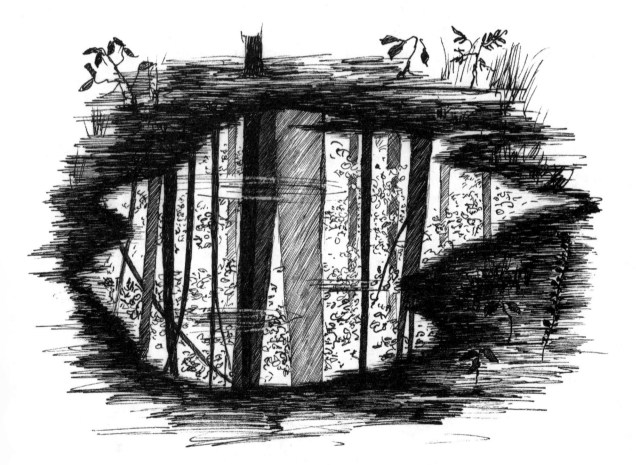

the Earth's energy rising upward through the healer's body and then flowing out through the heart, where love adds an essential ingredient for change. We are not healed by the heavens, much as we are inspired by them. Admire their beauty and understand that they are a part of one integrated complete environment, supporting all life forms. Do not forget that healing is done from the Earth and via the heart. Remember that people flow up and down simultaneously and relate to nature from both ends of their bodies. Health requires a good, strong and complete energy flow which moves from Earth toward heaven—from one pole of the body to the other pole of the body.

Nature is one. We are living in a fine place. It is our business to become healthy by regaining our energy flow in relationship to our environment, flowing from one end of our potential to the other.

10. Energy Anatomy

The energy of life is the bedrock of reality. Anatomy and psychology
are two different scholarly perspectives from which to view the
energy of life. When this energy manifests as matter, we call it the
physical body. When we feel the movement of the energy, we call
it emotion. When we pay attention to its content, we call it thought.

The human being is a flowing cylinder-shaped system of energy
that connects at its bottom to the energy of the Earth.

The principal energy function of the feet and legs is to access the
Earth's energy. This is done by connecting the person to the Earth
and then spontaneously drawing the Earth's energy upward
through the body. Under natural conditions, people walk without

shoes or with little foot covering. When this occurs, the feet, and especially the toes, are used in a dynamic and vigorous way that easily pumps energy upwards. It is not that shoes prevent this, but the constraining shape of most shoes prevent this. In addition, having learned to walk in such shoes usually immobilizes the natural form of feet and reduces the movement of the foot muscles and connective tissue.

Even though somewhat reduced in "civilized" people, the Earth's energy still flows upwards through the feet and legs. Once the Earth's energy reaches the bottom of the spine, it is relayed upwards through a series of seven vortices of energy which are called chakras. This is a Sanskrit word with no English equivalent. Each chakra's task is to create and then distribute the appropriate frequency of energy to all nearby body parts. As energy is consciousness, each chakra is characterized by a certain form of intelligence. Look at the illustrations entitled Chakras in a Mature Adult; they will help you understand the rest of the chapter.

Chakras are not objects. They are not things. They are movements in the flow of human energy, just as a whirlpool is a movement in the flow of a river. They form the "topographical map" of human energy. There is nothing arcane or mysterious about them—they are as ordinary as a grocery cart, as much a part of every person as the heart or stomach. As energy is life itself, it must have the capacity to do life's specialized functions. Consequently, each chakra is distinctly different from each other chakra in its location and its frequency. Going upward from seat to head the frequency of the chakras get successively higher, except for the second chakra.

Each chakra flows out of the spinal cord and extends both forwards and backwards to form two cones or vortices of energy, one at the front of the body and one at the back. The first and seventh chakras are somewhat different, as they originate from the top and bottom of the spine and form only one cone of energy movement each. They form intake and outflow valves for the body at the bottom of the torso and top of the head. All seven chakras

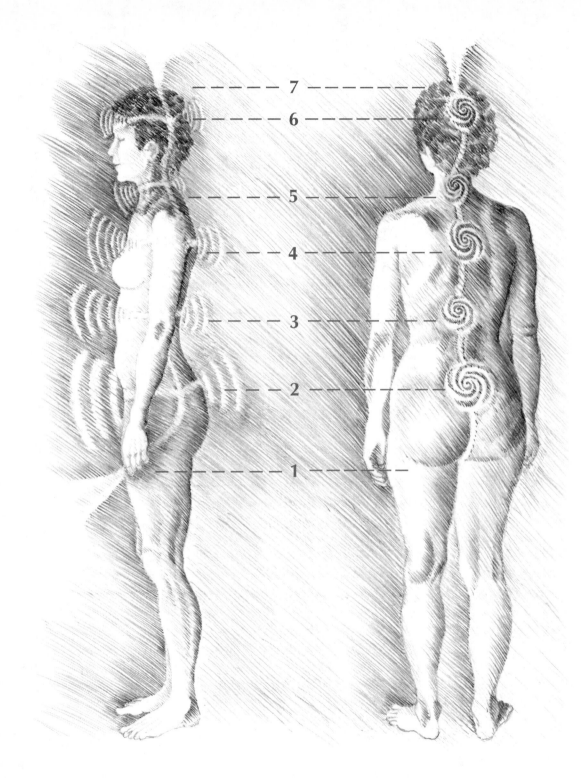

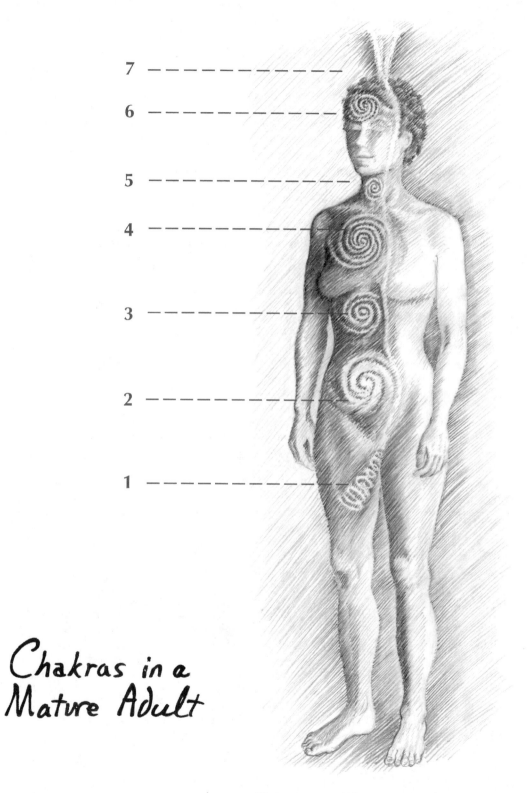

7 – – – – – – – – – –

6 – – – – – – – – – –

5 – – – – – – – – – –

4 – – – – – – – – – –

3 – – – – – – – – – –

2 – – – – – – – – – –

1 – – – – – – – – – –

Chakras in a
Mature Adult

flow past the surface of the physical body, as human energy is not limited to that area of the person bounded by the skin.

The first of these chakras is at the very bottom of the pelvis. Its primary purpose is to connect the person to the Earth—to life. It supplies the body with energy. The size and shape of a person's first chakra determines his basic attitudes toward staying alive and towards mating. These attitudes are only secondarily determined by thoughts or socially acquired values.

The energy flows upward from the first chakra and arrives at the second chakra, which is located below the waistline. Again the frequency of the energy is changed by being whirled about in this

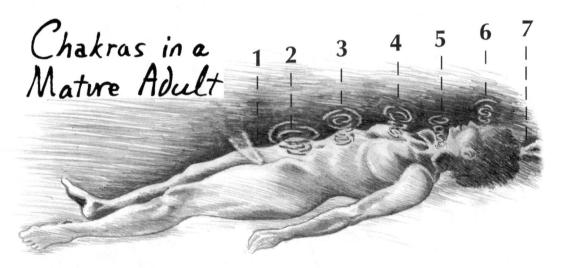

Chakras in a Mature Adult

1 2 3 4 5 6 7

chakra. For the purposes of the pelvis and its contents, the frequency of the energy is lowered. It is then distributed to the pelvic organs. In the first year of life the energy in this part of the infant's body acquires a rhythm and motion in response to the mother's pelvic energy. This acquired pattern of energy flow generally lasts a lifetime and becomes that person's basic attitude towards other people. Why? Because it was the mother's basic attitude towards the baby. It was experienced and acquired in this time before the child was old enough to think. Consequently, as important as this is to one's behavior, people generally have no awareness of this general attitude in themselves. It is the background to thought and feeling. This background makes it possible to be calm or not, thus coloring all else that occurs in a life.

The energy then rises to the third chakra, which is centered at the solar plexus. The third chakra raises the frequency of the energy so that it is appropriate for the needs of the organs in this area: liver, gall bladder, stomach, pancreas, spleen and diaphragm. These organs vibrate at the same frequency of energy that is used for logical or rational thinking. As the rational thoughts of people are generated by the third chakra, the disorders of these thoughts, or neuroses, inhere in this area. The organs on the left side of the third chakra are easily troubled by loneliness and sadness. The organs on the right struggle with anger and the desire to control life excessively. Much human misery is the result of energy disorders in this area which are generally caused by early childhood responses to one's parents. These energy disorders also play a determining role in causing physical disease. The bulk of presentations to physicians and counselors are problems of the third chakra area.

As the energy rises yet again, upward through the diaphragm and into the thoracic cavity, it is transformed into a still higher frequency by the fourth chakra. This energy is used by the heart and lungs. It has reached a high enough frequency to do great things. It is the energy of love. It can be used to take certain ordinary behaviors and form them into events that can make one's own and others' lives happy and healthy. Love is the energy that improves life. Love, the energy from a healthy and open fourth chakra, is the absolute precondition for healing. There is nothing vague or mystical about love. It is a precise frequency of human energy.

From here the energy rises upward until it reaches the fifth chakra, which is in the throat. At the fifth chakra, the frequency of energy is for the purposes of communication, creativity and balance. At this location all the polar aspects of the self are balanced: masculine versus feminine, conscious versus unconscious, and so forth. In addition, biochemical balancing takes place here. The organs of the throat and mouth are, of course, energized by the fifth chakra. Interestingly, their health is strongly affected by one's engaging in honest or less–than–honest expression. Dishonest or inhibited expression skews the energy flow at the throat. This in turn affects the other functions of the fifth chakra. The entire person is consequently affected by his or her habitual style of self-expression, since the fifth chakra is central in all balancing. This principle is important in maintaining one's health and is often the key to restoring health in those suffering with thyroid disorders.

From the fifth chakra, the energy rises to the middle of the forehead, where it is elevated in frequency by the sixth chakra, sometimes called the "third eye." Indeed, the sixth chakra is a perceptual "organ." It is that location in the flow of human energy which has the potential for knowing beyond the limits of the ordinary. Many are drawn to develop the capacities of the sixth chakra, to glimpse into the future. This is not power. Health is true power. Only health makes love possible, and health begins by developing the first chakra, the connection to the Earth.

At the very top of the head is the seventh and last of the chakras. Functioning like a chimney, it provides an upward vent for the linear flow of the person's energy. A competent healer must extend energy as high above the head as s/he can reach down through his or her feet. This will increase his or her power.

Power can be defined as the capacity to move a given volume of energy along the length of the body in a given time period. Such power alone cannot heal people, but when combined with love, it can. Assuming the healer, teacher or parent has an open heart, the amount of her power potentiates her love.

You must understand that energy is intelligence, and that other than the second chakra, each chakra creates successively higher frequencies of energy and thus higher intelligence (not intellect) than the chakra beneath. In this way higher and higher levels of consequent behavior become possible, but only if the entire system of energy is healthy and properly connected to the Earth.

This elegant system provides us with all of the possibilities and all of the limitations that comprise our lives. The goal of healing is to improve energy flow. The goal of improved energy flow is improving one's life. The goal of improving one's life is improving life for others.

11. Anger and Forgiveness

Anger is the most common cause of human unhappiness and poor health. Whether it takes the form of rage or resentment, whether it is expressed aloud or thought silently to oneself, whether it is conscious or unconscious, it is anger that sickens the greatest number of people. Anger is the most ignored cause of physical disease and the least successfully treated of psychological symptoms.

Anger cannot be eliminated by instruction, expression, compensation or repression. These are the usual ways in which we try to escape anger's discomfort. The transformation of anger into love is its only cure. Working with this principle must be the bedrock of the practice of healing, as so many psychological and physical symptoms are derived from anger, whether the causative event is recent or long past.

This is a difficult topic to write about, as there are no words in the English language that describe the process of transforming negative feelings into love. The word "forgive" approaches this, but in conventional usage this word is lost in a mire of legalism and the belief that either finding another guilty or declaring him free of responsibility is somehow significant. It is not. Neither the life of the judged nor that of those who judge is are improved by engaging in that process.

The word "forgive" is conventionally used to mean that, in spite of the other's wrongdoing against us, we release him from accountability. This will not improve health or happiness. Forgiving is not letting the other person off the hook; it is letting oneself off the hook (of anger). To forgive is to transform anger into love; this is the only useful definition.

Forgiving might follow this simple scenario: after exploring a particular grudge that the patient holds against another person, the healer proposes that s/he forgive that person. The patient will probably protest. The healer then gently asserts that there is no other way in which the patient can come to feel good and to be healthy. The patient then lies or sits, ideally on the ground, and the healer sits with the patient and opens his or her own heart. This creates appropriate modeling of energy and support for the needed change in the patient's heart. Regarding the patient with love, the healer asks him or her to pay attention to the center of his or her own chest, his fourth chakra. When s/he does this it begins to expand with energy, readying him or her to forgive, as the energy emanating from the middle of the chest is love. Then the healer could instruct the patient to imagine the person at whom he is angry. This brings two disparate elements together: an open heart and the object of the patient's anger. An open heart is in a state of love. Because no one can do two opposite acts at the same time, placing anger in love's presence is the beginning of forgiving.

The next step, which may be done then or at a second meeting, is to say the words," I forgive you" to the object of that person's anger, as if the words were coming out of the heart and not out of the mouth. The success of this process is dependent to a great extent on the healer's ability to maintain an open heart while the patient is trying to do this. If the healer does, the environment, that is the energy around the patient, is filled with love and the patient has the optimal conditions within which to succeed.

It is important to include bitterness, resentment, hatred, irritation, petulance, argumentativeness, grouchiness, sulkiness and contempt under the title of anger. These variations of anger sicken the body and destroy happiness in much the same way as outright anger. They also can be successfully resolved only by forgiveness, followed by forming a new emotional habit. Different kinds of anger affect specific organs and habits of responding to life's difficulties. For example, bitterness, an habitual angry belief that one is unfairly burdened, affects the kidneys. Hatred, on the other hand, effects the colon and is less conscious.

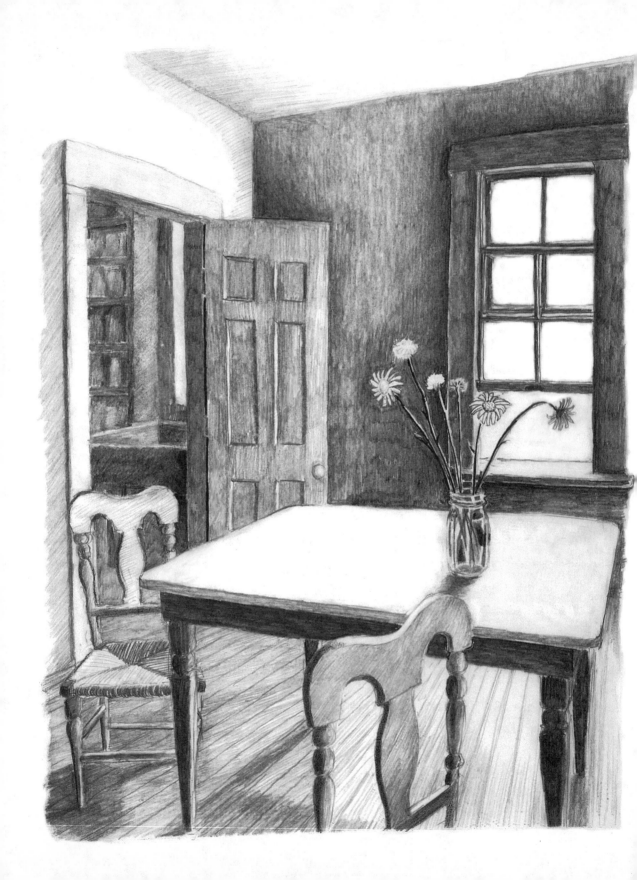

A large part of people's lives is driven by proving that one is worthy, redeeming oneself for prior wrongdoing, vindicating oneself, or getting revenge. The list is endless. There are moments of personal triumph when one imagines that closure has occurred, only to find later on that other feelings of incompletion still drive one's behavior. There is only one way of getting the peace that accompanies being finished with hurt, wrong, sleight or unfairness: to forgive the person or persons responsible for one's plight. This may be as intimate as forgiving a cruel parent or as distant as forgiving a political figure.

Only forgiveness transforms anger.

12. Fear

There is a prejudice in our society against acknowledging that one is afraid or even knowing that one is afraid. We replace the word fear with other words like anxiety, nervousness and tension. These euphemisms confuse people so that some are not certain whether they are frightened or not. If they do not clearly identify their discomfort, they cannot take the appropriate action to relieve it. This is of major importance, as fear is an emergency state. If it endures, it detracts considerably from health.

Fear also prevents people from loving. Fear and love are mutually exclusive states. In fear the heart energy, that is the fourth chakra, is contracted. Fear keeps us from our birthright of love, our highest potential. It is love that can make life good—make us happy and content.

Why is fear so common? Because children are raised by frightened or frightening parents. To blame these parents accomplishes nothing: they are merely people and were quite recently children with parents like themselves.

Still, fearfulness is learned quickly. It then stays fixed in the pattern of a person's energy flow, providing a response that occurs as if it were a reflex. In fear, one contracts. Obviously the superficial muscles tighten. Significantly, the diaphragm contracts upwards, all but severing the frightened person's energy connection with the Earth. In fear we are thus disconnected from the Earth, and consequently under-energized. If the fear lasts too long, we become ill.

Any time you become frightened, pause and do the standing exercises (see appendix). This will help you to literally reconnect to the Earth, your energy will flow again and fear will begin to change into comfort.

Although chronic fear can inhere in many places in a person's body, it is most frequently seen in the following four: heart, spleen, diaphragm and sixth chakra (the energy pattern of the forehead). The fear in each of these places is somewhat different.

A fearful heart lacks courage. A person with this limitation to the movement of energy collapses in the face of difficulty. A later chapter of this book deals with courage.

If the energy of the spleen does not flow in a healthy pattern, it creates a noisy internal experience of worry. Compulsively and repetitively trying to solve problems, or not being able to stop a melody or a phrase from repeating, are some of the typical experiences of a fearful energy pattern in the spleen.

If the energy flow through the diaphragm is inadequate, a person is subject to terror, a form of fear so extreme that it can be disabling.

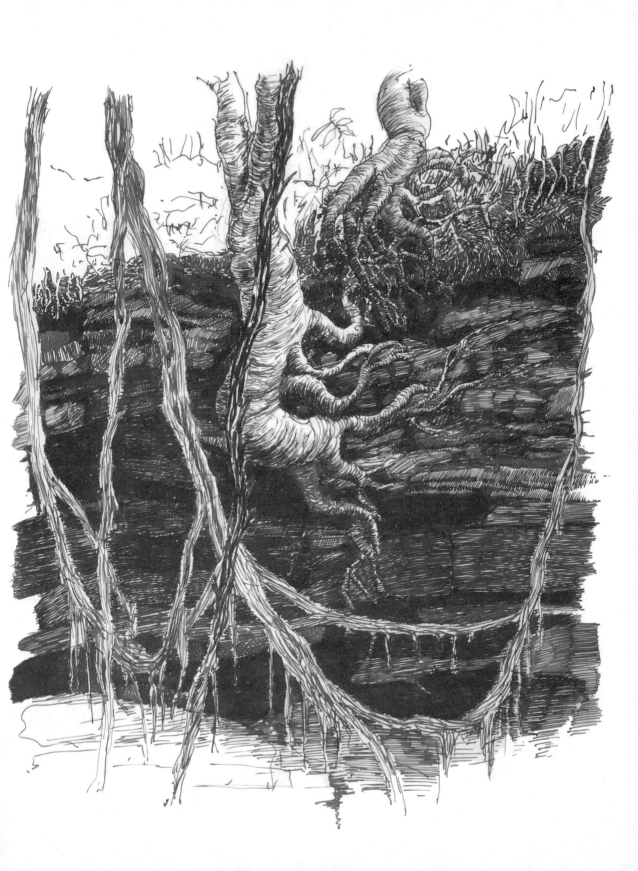

If these terror responses become attached to specific stimuli, such as small spaces or animals, they become phobias.

Should a child grow up in a family where he feels endangered (whether or not an outsider would say that this is objectively true), he develops a stance of wariness or mistrust. Mistrust is fear as an attitude, as a way of life. This takes the form of an oversized sixth chakra which is then misused as if it were a sensing device to scan for danger.

Each of these conditions can be healed in a general sense. A skilled healer can mediate the reorganization of spleen, heart, diaphragm or sixth chakra and help the process of being unafraid to begin. The patient must then commit to a daily regimen of interacting with the Earth. As one engages attentively and earnestly with the Earth, through the exercises in the appendix or by another means, the body releases waste energy and takes on healthy Earth energy. Over time one becomes healthier and less fearful (they go together).

Many can have the experience of a deep internal realization that they are safe, as they do have a mother, the great mother, the Earth, who is always present and will respond to their needs. If such a realization occurs, one will have precious little fear.

Fearfulness is a continual emergency state that stresses the person so badly as to ultimately cause destruction of bodily tissue. Reducing or eliminating fear is in many cases the solution to physical or psychological disease.

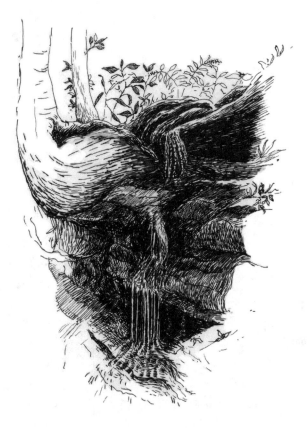

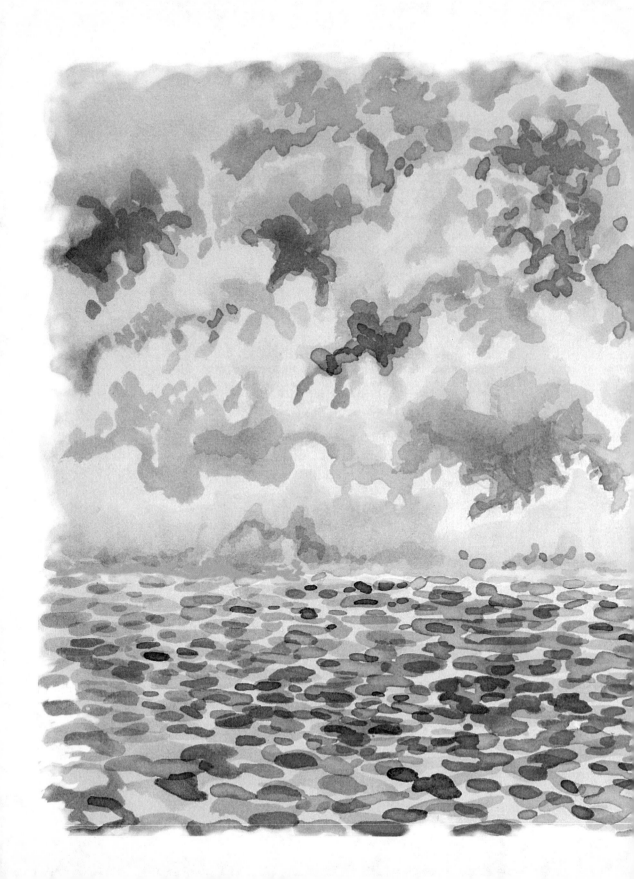

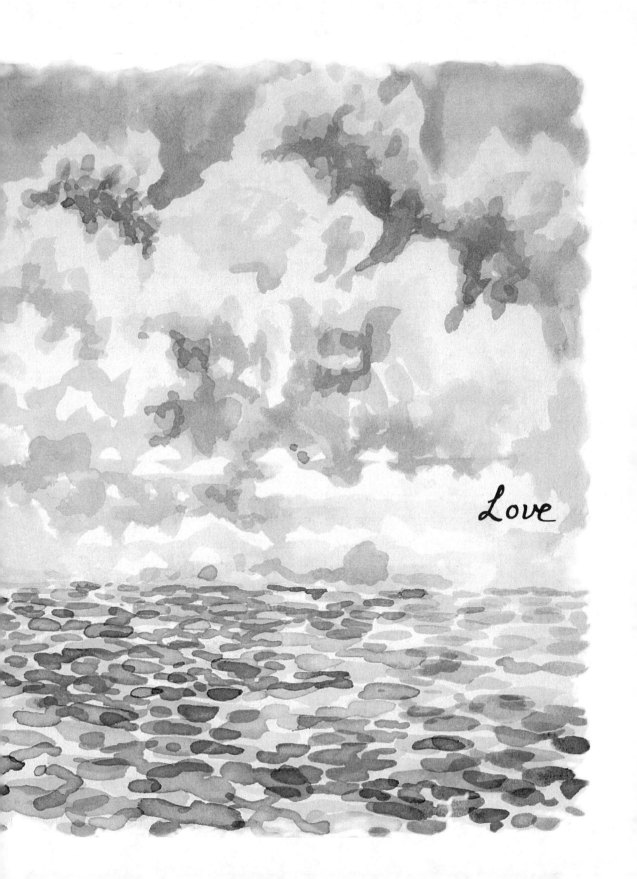

Love

13. Love and Courage

Love is the specific frequency of energy generated by a healthy and open heart or fourth chakra. It is not the other experiences that are often called love, such as sexual attraction, aesthetic appeal, emotional attachment, familial obligation or patriotism. *Love is the specific frequency of energy generated by a healthy and open fourth chakra.* All people respond to this energy, although they may not be able to understand or articulate their experience.

In the presence of a loving other, a person can exceed his usual limitations. When love is combined with instruction, learning occurs in ways otherwise not possible. When love is combined with limit setting, the misbehaving person may well comply. When love is combined with healing procedures, whether conventional or alternative, the patient can heal.

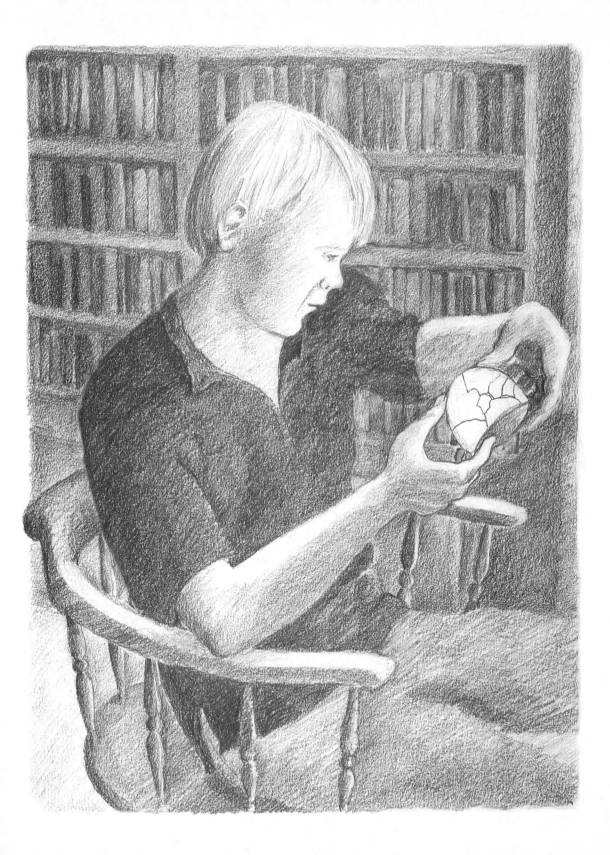

Love is a part of human energy and intelligence that supersedes reason. Its conclusions are not limited by logic. Its concern is not self-centered, but selfless. Love is the source of the answers to disease and meaninglessness.

The heart is the site where one experiences courage (the French word coeur means heart). Courage is not, as the media suggest, ignoring one's fear in order to aggressively encounter others. "Courage" on the battlefield is not courage at all; it is only youthful folly, and may even be an absence of love for self and other, a lack of knowledge that we are all connected, that we rise and fall together.

True courage is the capacity to buoyantly continue on while engaged in meaningful activity. A less than competent heart chakra contracts into fearfulness or disappointment, which prevents one from enduring under difficult circumstances.

Where does the energy of courage come from? Around the fourth chakra there is a last ring of energy that expands when one is faced with duress. In a healthy person this is present. In a person who has been raised by either one or both parents who lacked courage, it does not develop appropriately. Without this capacity for expansion of the heart's energy, one cannot respond adequately to extremely demanding or frightening moments. This is an aspect of human energy that does not mature without a model during a sensitive period of development (approximately four years of age).

What can be done later on? A fine healer can stand between the patient and the energy of nature and mediate courage for this patient. The patient must then engage in a series of daily exercises to use this additional heart energy. These may range from vigorous exercise to generosity.

The healing of the heart is of central importance to both prevention and remediation of disease. To wait for the symptoms of heart disease before healing the heart is absurd. This is because only an adequate heart can "grow" the person into a mature adult who is able to accept the responsibilities of protecting the family and doing good works. The person without sufficient energy in his heart cannot protect and nurture children or Earth. Work must generate goodness for others; this is the only means to success for the world. That is why one needs the courage to work well in the face of obstacles.

Without a healthy fourth chakra one is not a healthy person. But a healthy fourth chakra cannot exist without a healthy first chakra to supply it with sufficient energy. Thus the first task in healing the heart is going to the Earth (see appendix of exercises), and learning to access its energy.

Healers' hearts must be strong and willing to expand. A fearful or easily tired healer could not perform well. The loving healer is nourishing and encouraging for the hearts of all those about him or her even without doing formal healings. This is because the presence of a large, courageous heart continuously evokes imitative responses from others' hearts.

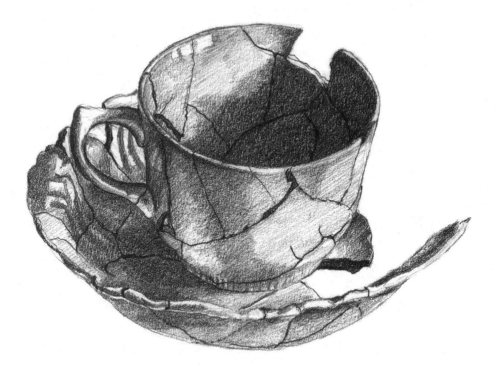

14. Healing Parents

Love is often absent in the lives of parents and their children. What is referred to as love in this situation is often that fierce attachment that parents have to their offspring. This attachment and the watchfulness that goes with it keep children alive and safe. It provides the most meaningful activity in most people's lives. No wonder many people call this love, as little else they have experienced matches this for intensity and meaning—but it is other than love.

The ways in which parents' own lives are limited will, of course, characterize their parenting of their children. No matter how much they wish to do otherwise, the nature of their energy will influence their parenting. For a short period of time they can use their will and do better, but such efforts soon collapse. Parents are merely people. They are their energy, and their energy, in many cases, is less than optimal.

Most parents do their best. They parent to the limit of their capacity, but none can exceed this. It is not possible. If they are fearful, for example, it is an expression of the configuration of their energy, and only healing can change this and help them towards better parenting.

Healing parents of young children must be a priority for all healers. If parents are healed they become better parents and their children will consequently have better lives. In healing parents the children are also healed. Why is this? Children, especially young children, live alongside the energy of their parents. The parent's energy is the most significant part of the children's environment. They are greatly responsive to this parental energy-environment, thriving if it is healthy, suffering if it is not.

If it is the healer's goal to improve the world, then it must be done by strategically choosing his patients. To heal a parent of young children improves the future of a family. The children of that family then become better adults. All people will then have a better future.

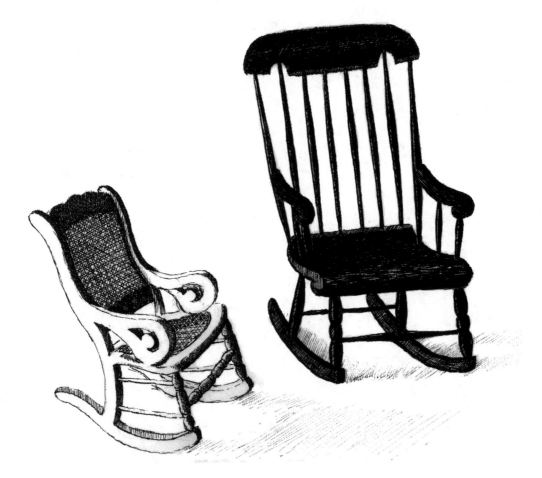

15. Patience

Patience, when authentic, flows from the energy of the heart. When unauthentic, it is merely endurance or waiting until a frustration passes. Often people are angry, irritated or bored while they wait for one another. True patience, however, is waiting with an open heart, an expanded fourth chakra, while the other takes the time needed to accomplish a task. Under these conditions, waiting is without stress.

Doing almost any task while aided by another's presence and attention increases one's efficiency and even one's ability. This often allows one to perform at a higher level than would be possible by oneself. To do a task with another person whose heart is patiently open adds further to one's ability and performance .

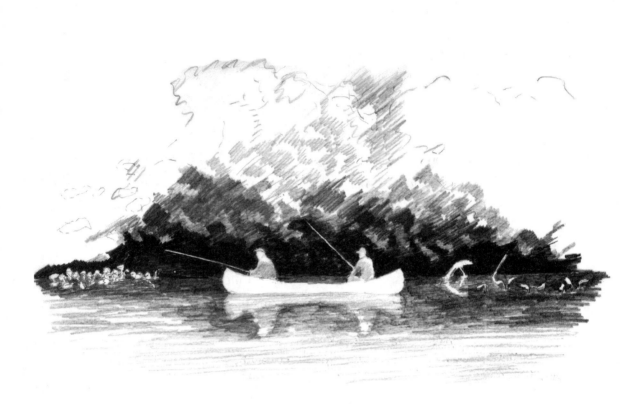

Patience is the ultimate facilitative skill. Patience is the behavior of parents that can evoke excellence from otherwise ordinary children. Patience is an essential tool for healers. In fact, the healer who is impatient is only pretending to do healing.

Patience is the principal gift that teachers can bring to students. Each student will take however long s/he must in order to learn the next lesson; but if that time is filled with loving energy, his or her efforts will be supported and his or her learning capacity nourished. However ungifted the student may be at a task, there will be no loss of esteem as s/he strives to succeed.

With patience, waiting can be a productive activity. This is quite the opposite of what most people believe. Someone who has mastered patience approaches the line at the bank teller's window and thinks "Oh, an opportunity. There is much loving to be done here."

Patience, waiting in love, is done with the energy of a healthy open fourth chakra.

16. Gentleness

Gentleness is the spontaneous quality of touch that inheres in all people as they hold infants. Gentleness is not only tender but supportive as well. Without support the baby would fall. Gentleness exists in this primal interaction because it protects life. So it is apparent that gentleness is a basic human attribute. If this is so, there should be much gentleness among people. Why then is there so much of its opposite? Because this natural and spontaneous impulse can be inhibited by the experience of unkind treatment.

The gentle touch may be physical or not. When people are gently treated they become civil and calm. When people are harshly treated, they contract with fear or anger. These two emotions erode their bodies and corrupt their relationships with others. The gently-treated child knows love as a daily tactile and auditory experience. S/he then behaves the same way to others. S/he can relax into growth and learning. The harshly-treated child becomes habitually angry or chronically sad.

Gentleness is one of the most needed additions to social custom, as the stresses of urban living leave many people in a chronic state of alertness. Continual alertness causes serious loss of quality of life and is a major precursor to illness. It requires gentleness to soothe this away and return people to calmness.

If a marriage is characterized by gentleness, problems have little power to seriously upset the spouses. Without gentleness, marriages easily become places of struggle and competition, leaving husbands and wives unfulfilled and bitter.

Gentleness is one of the behaviors that can express love's energy. It must be mastered by those who wish to be healers, as it is a necessary means to the other person's healing and learning. It does not matter what career role the healer has.

Gentleness is touching the other with loving support as if they were an infant.

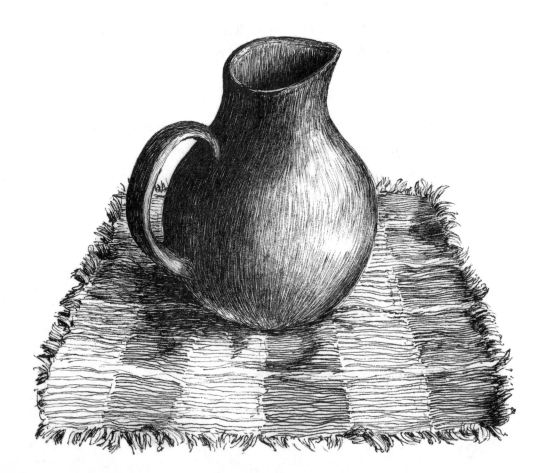

17. Kindness

Kindness is the inherent response of a healthy adult to a child in need. It is a reflex. Like all other reflexes, it protects life.

When parents are faced with their children's needs, whether hunger or pain, they respond spontaneously. If this is not experienced frequently in childhood it will only be reflexive in response to small children. If it is experienced frequently in childhood, the reflex of kindness also operates in response to adults in need.

When a kind person interacts with someone in need, s/he spontaneously orients to that need. Sometimes the kind response is words and sometimes not; sometimes it is a solution to a problem, but more often not. Most kindnesses are small in scale. Ideally this

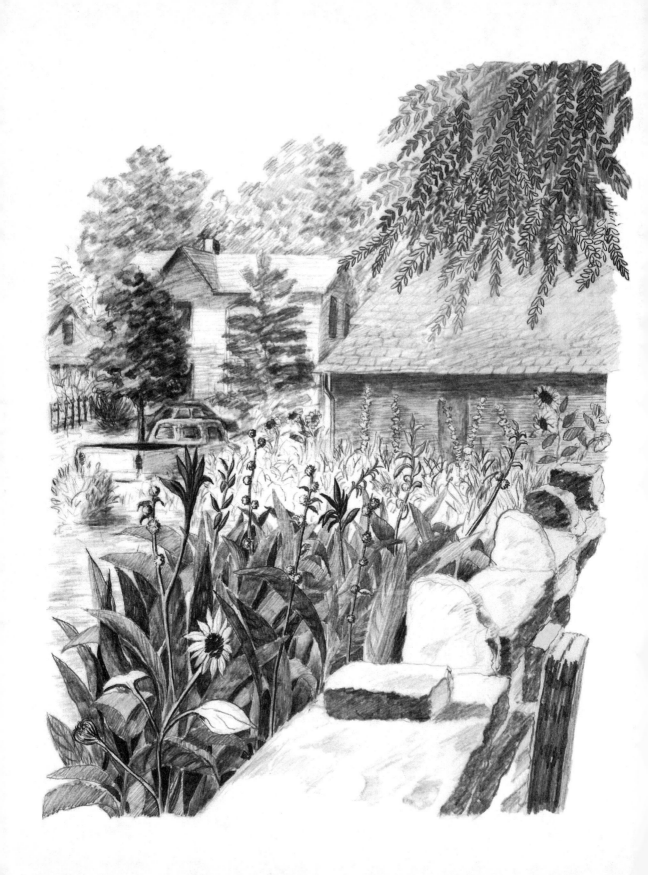

is an exchange of energy from the heart, formed into a kind act—a smile, a touch or a sympathetic sound.

When kind behavior is done while one's body flows with ample energy and one's heart is open, kindness then becomes a healing act. The recipient of such kindness can emerge changed for the better, with improved energy flow and new possibilities. They may not understand what has happened; some may have scarcely paid attention to the event—still, they will have been enhanced.

Acting kindly can improve your community. If your social interactions are kind, many people will respond to this light and loving touch. Acting kindly and doing so with an open heart is one way to be an authentic healer without ever conducting "formal" healings.

18. Generosity

Generosity is giving freely without fear of personal loss. This is difficult in a society that imagines that giving results in a reduction of one's wealth. But wealth is not, nor ever has been, financial assets. Wealth is energy.

To convey nature's energy is to be alive. To convey it in large amounts is to experience wealth, as the movement of that energy through a person causes feelings of happiness, competence, power, confidence and pleasure. The only thing a healer or anyone can do with this energy is to give it away. It can not be retained. The moment one holds back, one loses both pleasure and vigor. This is because holding back words or actions requires tightening one's body.

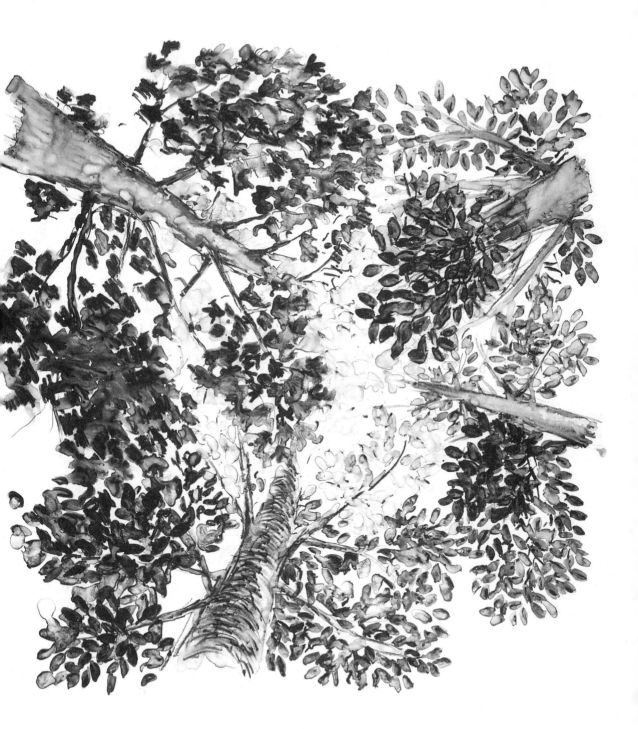

Giving labor, joy or love is never giving something of yours away. It is moving nature's energy through yourself and on to the next person, while enjoying the pleasant sensations of its passage. In fact, there is no giving and no receiving. These two words are linguistic conventions that fit within the structure of logic, but fail to capture the true nature of reality.

Generosity simultaneously feeds giver and receiver with the same energy. The economics of energy are different than accounting would predict. When one gives from the heart, the gift is carried lovingly to the other by the heart's energy while simultaneously nourishing the giver with love. Many people have had this experience, although it defies ordinary logic.

As one opens the heart in generosity, love flows outward and inward in one movement. Two people join in a moment of shared energy flow, initiated by the one who knows the secret of generosity.

19. Appropriate Social Behavior

Appropriate social behavior, ordinary conduct that benefits others, is the necessary social background for healing. As we are social animals, the energy generated by others becomes part of the environment in which we live. This is literally so. Appropriate behaviors that improve your environment, and hence your life, may include moments of consideration, warmth, self-restraint and mannerliness in an ordinary day.

These appropriate behaviors, which feel good to do and good to receive, are the building blocks of a healthy community. They create internal feelings of safety, order and comfort. These simple good behaviors will make everyone feel safe. If there is no general feeling of safety, there is little to be gained from healing, as a feeling of safety allows people to relax. Without relaxation the body spends its energy readying for flight or fight. With relaxation this same energy can be used to regenerate and to develop.

In places where socially appropriate behavior is rare, such as certain large cities, people are often frightened or angry, and easily become sick. If one does not ordinarily feel safe and relaxed in the presence of family and co–workers, one sickens. This has become so common that headaches and gastro-intestinal distress are considered normal by many people. These are the expressions of a frightened or angry body. If they occur often, more serious illness

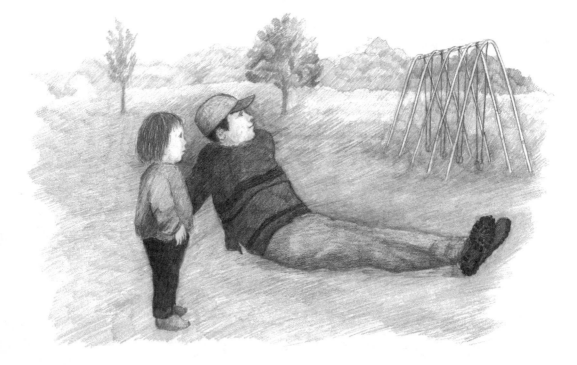

follows. Consequently, all of us will then suffer loss, as each person is part of our interdependent society.

Appropriate behavior must be fundamental social training received by all children. These lessons, like most childhood lessons, are learned mainly by imitating one's parents. If you teach your children to be indifferent or rude to others, they will cause harm to all, just as if they were adding toxic chemicals to the water supply. If you teach them, by your own behavior, a few formal manners, they will add to the well being of everyone they meet. Their contribution will be like that of a healthy tree whose vigor and beauty benefits all.

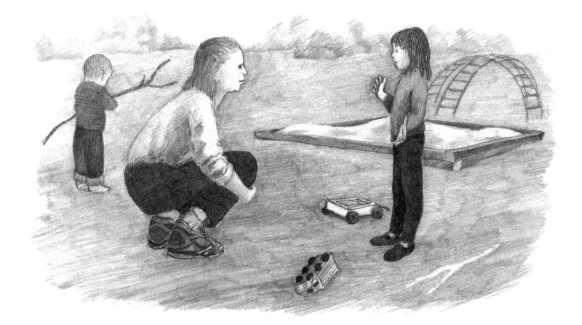

20. Delicacy

Delicacy is the most mature version of appropriate social behavior. It is a desire to save the other from unpleasantness, from noxious experience. It is a sensitivity to the unspoken needs of others not to be slighted or sickened. Delicacy is a hallmark of maturity. It is rarely seen in the young, as children are lost in their personal needs and wants. It is uncommon in young adults, as they are often driven by their appetites. The mature adult is finally freed from the insistence of internal demand, so it is possible for him to know that every interaction is of importance.

A delicate view of the other allows one not only a refined perception of the other's existence, but of the importance of that existence.

The mature adult understands that our social fabric is created by
the sum of all the interactions among people. He knows that harm
will occur to all of us if some must cringe from noxious stimulation.
Wanting a healthy society in which to live, he avoids behaving

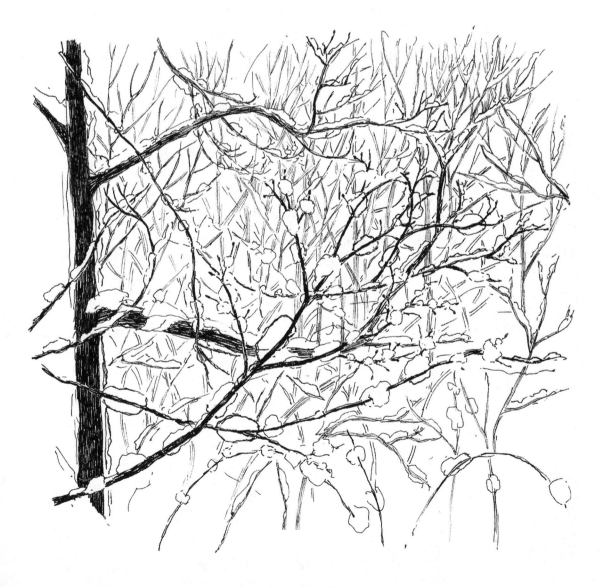

distastefully. Delicacy is essential to small tribes and primitive groups, or people who fully understand their interdependency. As a result they are conscientious in their choice of behavior. This may seem contradictory to a member of a large industrialized society, who imagines that s/he participates in the highest achievements of humanity. The opposite is pitifully so. Urbanization and industrialization have resulted in successive dehumanization. The challenge facing us is to regain a "primitive" sensibility and to practice that in daily life with friends and utter strangers alike.

Delicacy is a rarely considered idea at this time. But it is a way of conducting ourselves that can rescue us from urban harshness, with its attendant danger and despair. It is necessary for health, as its absence creates stress and stress causes disease.

If you want to expand into the full power and satisfaction of your humanity, this is one of the essential ingredients.

21. Tolerance

Tolerance is allowing the heart, the fourth chakra, to remain open in the presence of the unusual. Intolerance is closing the heart in the presence of the unusual.

Even if you have not yet spent much time paying attention to your heart, you may feel your response to another as a tightening or relaxing in your chest. When presented with behavior or appearance which varies from that with which you are familiar, you are facing a challenge to your heart. If you allow it to remain open, although the other person differs from you, your life will be enhanced. You will not have suffered the loss of energy and pleasure that accompanies tightening in the presence of difference.

As deviation from the mean is an unvarying principle of nature, you are certain to face peculiarity in others with frequency. To close your heart when in the presence of unusual appearance or behavior is to damn yourself to a life with a closed heart.

We live in a world populated by people who are not exactly like us. Keeping our hearts open in their presence makes us happier and healthier; closing our hearts brings impoverishment to all.

Certainly, tolerance is one of the essential traits in a successful marriage. All spouses differ from each other and many are not only intolerant of those differences, but engage in frequent battle about them. If a spouse practices seeing the other's differences without closing his or her heart, without tightening against the differences, the marriage will improve.

To become more tolerant can not be done intellectually. One must make a commitment to open one's heart, to stay soft in the face of novelty (see appendix of exercises). Tolerance is not merely fair or legally correct. It is healthy behavior.

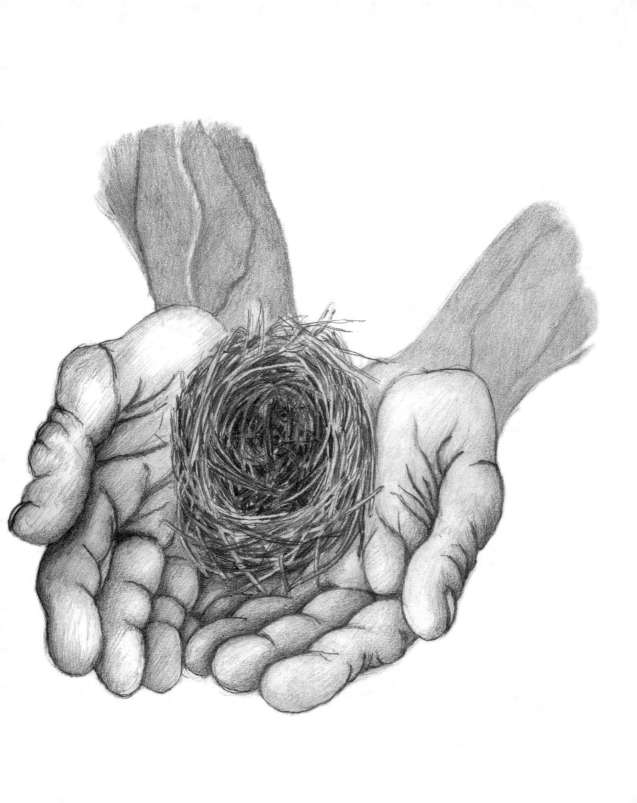

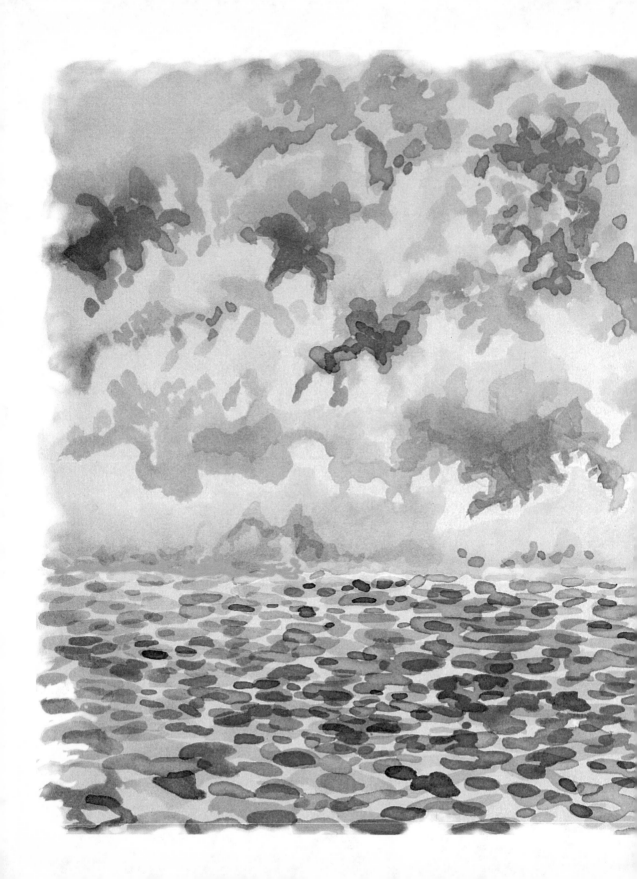

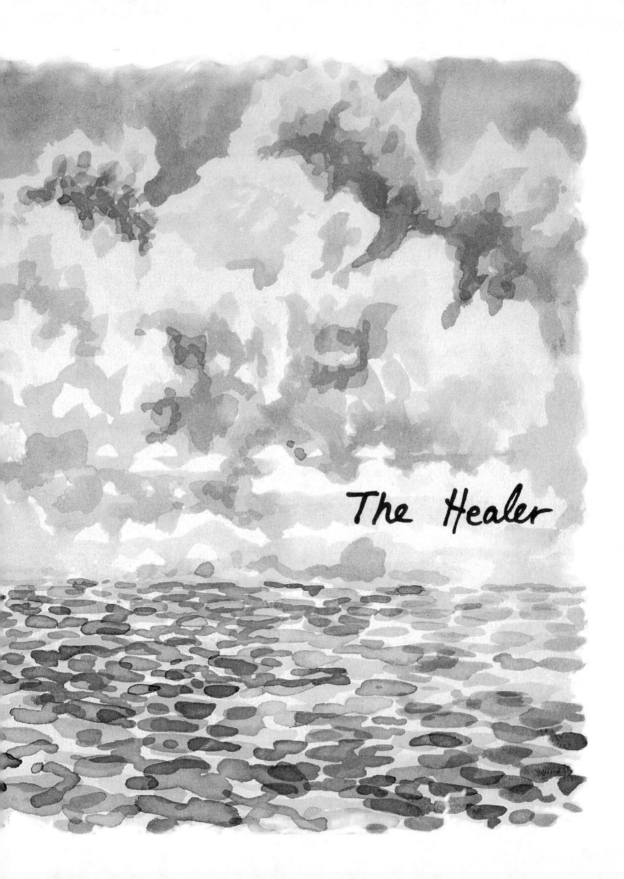

The Healer

22. Heart-Centeredness

The healer always works with his or her attention centered at the heart. This puts the healer in a loving state. If this heart–centeredness is lost, the healer relates to the patient from the intellect (which is one chakra too low to do healing). S/he falls back on the tools of analysis and reason, which have value, but do not heal people. In this state s/he easily becomes concerned with the other's demand for symptom relief. It is the heart that perceives past this demand and allows for the broadest view of the other's needs. Usually, analytical approaches to the other's pain have already been tried and have failed.

A symptom is just that—a symptom of something else—something unhealthy in the flow of the energy of that person. A symptom is a signal saying that there is a problem, but the symptom is not the problem per se. Nevertheless, most symptoms are unpleasant or unsightly. They must be, to get our attention. The intelligence of the heart responds to the greater need, the one indicated by the symptom. The intellect, by contrast, often seizes upon the obviousness of the symptom and the patient's desire to obliterate it.

The healer's heart fuels his or her generosity. Healers must be generous in order to allow the energy of nature to pass through themselves to others without trying to retain that energy. One cannot be authentically generous until one knows from experience that nature supplies limitless energy, that there is never a shortage, and that handing it on to another is not a personal loss. After experiencing this enough times, material generosity often develops spontaneously. Unselfishness is a sign of healthy good sense. It demonstrates the knowledge that objects fail to produce the meaningful outcomes of happiness, peacefulness or vigor.

It is the heart that generates gentleness, imitating a motherly touch. This is yet another of the needed ingredients for healing. Gentleness evokes sufficient trust from others to allow the acceptance of healing. The likelihood of successful healing without gentleness is low, because if the other is mistrustful or frightened, the healing will fail.

So the healer lives a heart-centered life. This means that much of the time s/he is paying attention to the heart, the fourth chakra. [Tap the center of your sternum and keep your attention where you feel that sensation. Do this for one or two minutes and see how your body and emotions change.] S/he does this while doing almost everything else—at the very same time. It turns life into a life colored by love, as attention to the heart continuously generates the exact frequency of human energy that calms and heals and gives hope and optimism.

A healer's presence is healing.

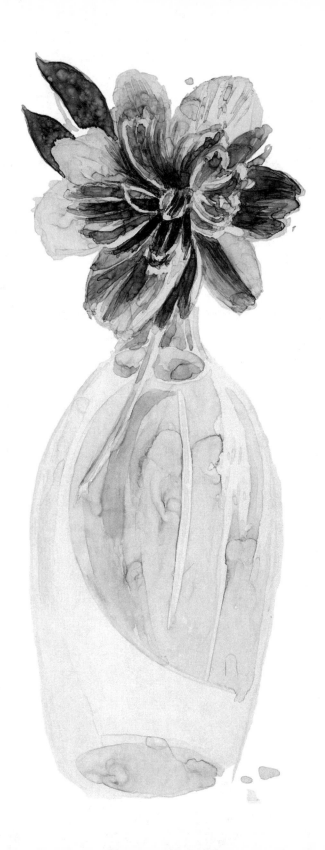

23. Balance and the Fifth Chakra

In the throat is the fifth energy vortex or fifth chakra. It spins at the frequency which is appropriate for communication, creativity and the balancing of a person's polar or contradictory qualities. For every trait we have, the potential for the opposite trait exists.

Much illness and unhappiness is the result of an imbalanced existence. This can be the imbalance of the right and left sides of the body, of the assertive and receptive modes of behavior, of immediate and long term concerns, or of sleeping and waking modes. If these or other polar aspects of one's life are unbalanced, the personality becomes exaggerated and begins to lack compensatory abilities. Ultimately this will cause exaggerated behavior as well as physical disease. This is a vicious circle as exaggerated behavior further exacerbates the lack of balance in the flow of one's energy. Imbalance leads to even greater imbalance.

Of all the chakras, only the fifth chakra provides a route for the body's energy to flow from the left side to the right side of the person. Through this place the balancing of energy, and hence the balancing of the person, can occur. However, to facilitate this balancing in the other, the healer must have a healthy fifth chakra.

The right and left sides of all people are different. Obviously each contains different organs. In addition, or because of that, the energy of each side is perceptibly different. The energy of the left side is slightly lower in frequency and is developed in response to one's mother's energy during the first year of life. The right side is slightly higher in frequency than the left and is developed in response to one's father's energy during the fourth to sixth years of life. To have an absent, sick, depressed, unwilling, mourning or alcoholic parent during either of these formative periods causes negative consequences in the formation of one's patterns of energy.

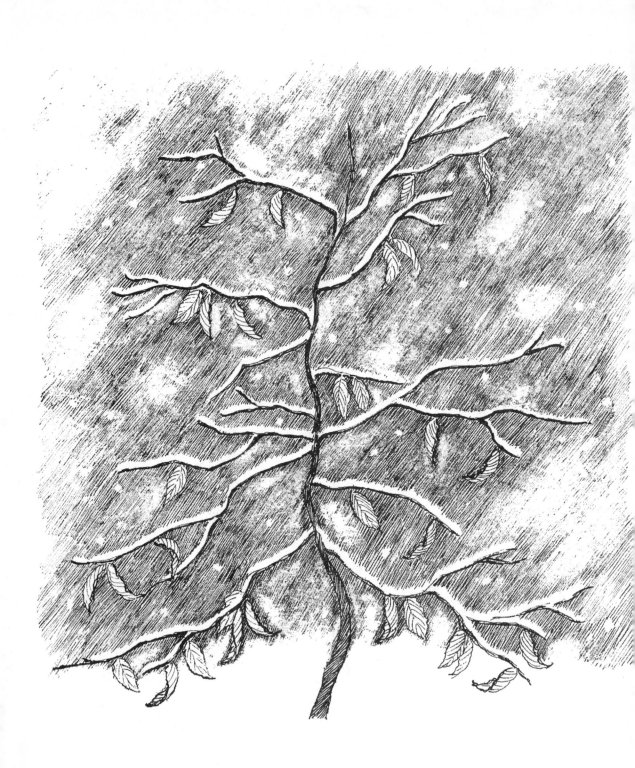

The energies of each side are different; thus the abilities generated by each are different. The right is more conscious and intentional. The left is more intuitive and more receptive. Both of these modes of behavior are necessary for a successful life. One is not superior to the other. They are two parts of a balanced existence.

Significantly, the left side has a tendency to be less conscious than the right side, but it is not unconscious. In highly developed people there is no unconsciousness; instead, they have access to the memories of their experiences and are able to think about them. Less well-developed people do not have such skill. The most extreme form of this is insightlessness. Insightless people have little ability to think about their own past experiences, and thus fail to understand human behavior, either their own or others.

Getting healthier almost always involves improving oneself by way of having new experiences. This not only requires the trait of insight, but the willingness to use it by actively paying attention to one's physical and emotional experience. So being healed by the Earth, whether or not via a healer, is not a passive process. It requires active engagement followed by a willingness to try new ways of living.

Those whose energy is impeded or disordered on the right side have lives characterized by impulsiveness and irresponsibility. As a result they bring disorder to their families and communities. These people end up receiving a great deal of attention from the legal and social service professions. Conversely, disorders of the energy of the left side fall into two general categories: chronic depression and insightlessness. Their physical, psychological and social sequelae typically are brought to the attention of the medical profession.

The fifth chakra is the fulcrum of balance. To use it well, to live a balanced life, requires attentive engagement with the Earth and active engagement with your experiences.

To heal or to avoid problems with the fifth chakra, avoid drugs (which cause bio-chemical imbalance); speak openly of your experiences (which helps you to be balanced through honest expression); and address any "extremism" or "one-sidedness" in your life, such as a prejudice, an unwillingness to engage with other than a certain group of people or an extreme and limiting belief system.

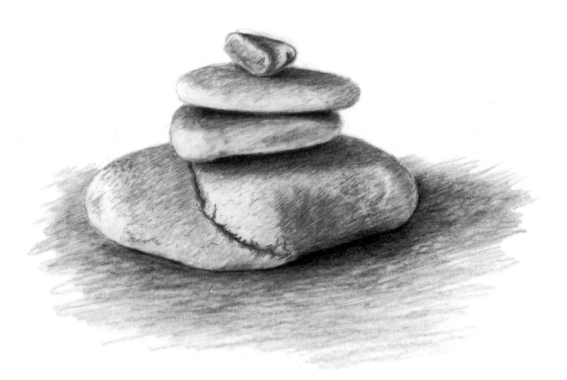

24. Becoming a Healer

The would–be healer, much like an athlete or an artist, will do best with a gift or talent to do this work. To acquire the skill of doing healing or hitting a baseball is simple. To do so at the level of expertise required for excellence requires effort and desire, gift or not.

To become a healer it is best to find a master, not a teacher. Although "master" is not a frequently used word in our culture, the distinction is important. One seeks a person who has mastered the challenges of healership. One then connects to the master through a relationship characterized by respect and hard work. When in the presence of the master, one's energy spontaneously imitates the superior organization of the master's energy. This spontaneous imitation of another's excellence is a common experience. Have you not felt more creative, witty or even graceful sharing activities with certain people?

One must also observe the energies of nature each day. This is the second opportunity to imitate mastery. In meditative attention to the Earth, trees and plants, one spontaneously imitates their energy and is improved by doing this.

If the would–be healer does this work earnestly each day and practices loving as well as connecting to the Earth, s/he will soon be ready to mediate healing from nature for others. To do this s/he would intentionally organize his or her own energy in the presence of this other person. This is done by first accessing the energy from the Earth through the feet into a strong flow through the body, and then opening the heart in love. In this optimal state the healer is a means through which nature's energy can pass to the person in need.

The energy of the healer and therefore the life of the healer must be orderly. The healer lives a simple life. Knowing that people are diurnal, s/he rises early. In order to keep his or her health and strength at a level that supports doing healing, s/he exercises out of doors each day. Only outdoor exercise moves enough of the Earth's energy through the body to strengthen and support it sufficiently for the work of life. In short, the healer is healthy. One who would conduct the energy of nature to another must provide a healthy vehicle for this process. A less than healthy healer would cause a reduction in the quality of the energy, much as a rusty pipe would reduce the quality of drinking water.

The healer carefully chooses which substances to put in his or her body, eating a simple diet and avoiding alcohol, tobacco and drugs. These all tax the body severely, especially the liver, kidneys and spleen, and so would reduce the healer's vitality.

The healer rarely gets angry. Knowing that anger is the principal cause of disease, s/he has given it up. This does not mean that s/he represses awareness of anger or suppresses its expression. S/he has

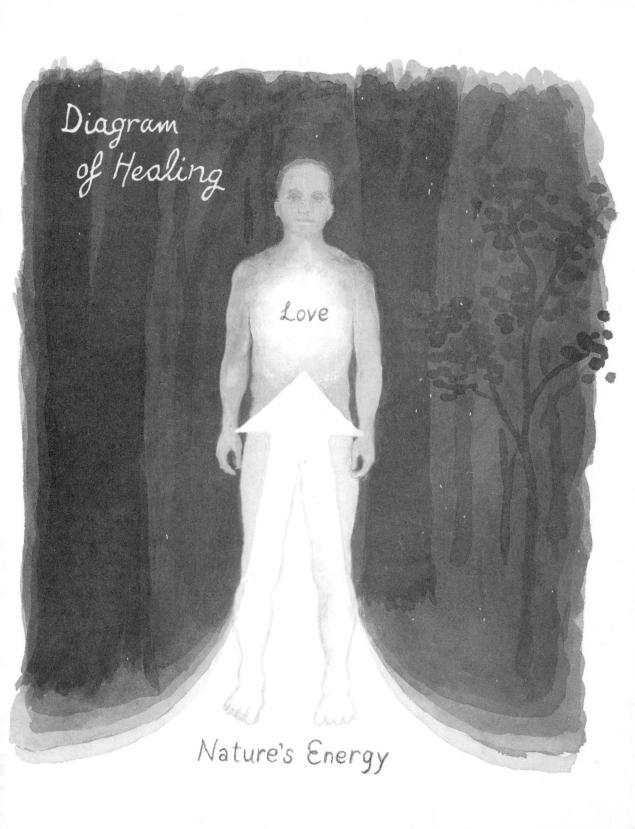

eliminated anger by systematically practicing forgiveness each time s/he has become angry. This has created a gentler way of responding to the unavoidable difficulties of daily life.

This method of retraining oneself from habitual anger into almost no anger requires first that one make a clear decision to change. The actual process then takes the form of gently interfering with one's (usually internal) anger. Upon hearing oneself mutter words of resentment or anger, one pauses and places a hand on the heart, then lightly says, "I don't want to be angry; I will be happy instead." This could happen fifty times a day in the beginning, but in a few months, anger will be infrequent. In six to nine months of this gentle practice, anger will be a rarity.

Healers are wise. This does not mean that they know secrets, rituals or obscure information. Wisdom is a great amount of common sense. How does this happen? It is the result of spending time each day connecting to the energy of the Earth. Wisdom is neither intellectual nor esoteric.

This calm and orderly style of life is deeply pleasant. It is also the means to profoundly rewarding work.

To be a healer is to be master of your own energy flow. If you do this, those who are in your presence will unconsciously imitate the superior level of your energy organization and find themselves improved.

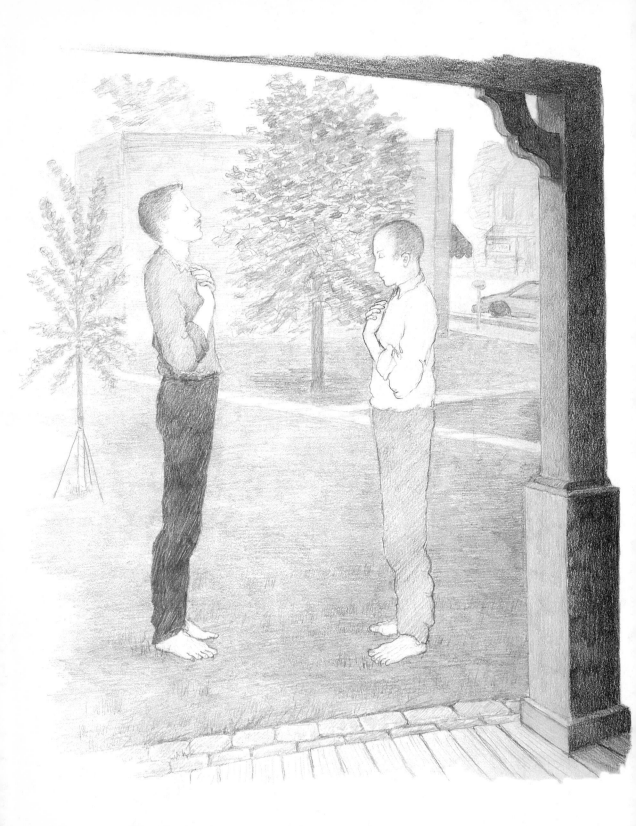

25. Healers Are Teachers

It is unlikely that healing will be fully successful if it is not accompanied by learning some type of new behavior that will support this new organization of energy. The problem that was just healed was partially caused by unhealthy behavior, whether in the form of thinking, feeling or doing. For example, a person with frequent headaches must learn to forgive, as headaches are usually caused by anger.

All healers are thus teachers of healthy behavior. They must be teachers in order to help others turn the healing into an improved life. The sort of teaching that results in changed behavior is usually experiential teaching—arranging a new experience for the other, not instructing the other. Imagine a person with chronic depression, which is an energy disorder of the left side of the body. To be successfully healed, the left side energy must be reorganized. Then the patient will have a normal pattern of energy flow. After this s/he must learn to behave vigorously or the healing is for naught. If you say "Now, you must do robust exercise every day," he or she will not, as a lifetime of experience has clearly demonstrated that s/he cannot. The healer must arrange for this person to discover his or her changed capacities. The beginning of this might be as simple as taking a walk together.

Experiential learning, doing something one has never done before, can result in changed behavior, thoughts and feelings. It is effective because we easily trust our experience, while tending to mistrust second hand information.

There are many things that cannot be learned from instruction. You cannot learn to dance by reading a book; you cannot learn to recognize a new scent from a lecture; you cannot learn joy from a direction manual. All three, however, can be learned by experience, especially in the company of someone who already is successful doing one of these.

Intellectual learning, as opposed to experiential learning, is the memorizing, reciting and reorganizing of information. It is often the principal means and end product of our schools. Intellectual learning, as opposed to experiential learning, will not result in healing or becoming healthier.

The healer must listen carefully as the patient presents the problem that precedes the healing. When the healing is over, the healer then proposes a relevant learning experience. This is an invitation to try something novel and indicated by the problem. This learning experience takes advantage of the potential of the reorganized energy accomplished by the healing. It involves the patient in healthy action that was absent or insufficient before the healing.

For example, someone has told the healer of being depressed. The healer then does a simple and natural healing. Then, taking the patient by the hand, s/he leads him to doing a small kindness for some other person— a smile, a quiet word, a bit of help.

Often, however, the patient will view the proposed new activity as a danger or problem. This is because all people are unconsciously organized to fend off change. Avoiding debate or excessive explanation, the healer might gently say "Stand here with me on the grass and pay attention to the sensations of your feet." Then s/he stands quietly with the patient, making the patient's success more likely by the addition of a second person's calm energy. This is like the work of an ideal parent or teacher, inviting a child to try something new, explaining how to begin and then calmly supporting the endeavor by presence and good will.

Telling a cigarette smoker that s/he must stop because smoking causes emphysema will probably fail. This is an example of intellectual teaching. If it succeeds by frightening the patient, his or her fearful or resentful compliance will cause sickness in new ways. Instead, take the smoker outdoors and ask him or her to lie on the ground in order to cleanse the lungs by paying attention to the sensation of the back (lungs) against the ground. Afterward listen with an open heart as s/he explains how different s/he feels—how light and optimistic.

Words teach people new ideas.

Experiences teach people new behavior.

New behavior is more easily learned after healing.

26. Levels of Healing

There are a number of different ways to do healing, many of which are systematized as schools or methods of healing. There are also ways of healing that are folk ways from various cultures. Ways of doing healing can be arranged in a series of levels from least reorganizing of the patient's energy to most reorganizing, in other words, from least transforming to most transforming.

What is being described in this book is not a method or system of healing. It is the essence of healing—unadorned, authentic and acultural. It is a natural way to interact with our environment and to then mediate between nature and others with our love. Excellence in this irreducible form of healing could place it at the very highest levels of healing. With less skill one might perform at a lower level of healing.

At the bottom of this hierarchy of healing are the necessary behaviors that create the social environment—the background for successful healing. These are ways of conducting ourselves that create a safe and healthy community. They include warmth, mannerliness, offering assistance, consideration, social orderliness and lawfulness. If we behave in these ways regularly, we will promote feelings of safety and reassurance. Only if these conditions are present can people be relaxed enough to become healthy. The importance of this cannot be overlooked if you want health. The body of a person who lives in a stressful social environment, such as a large city, a dysfunctional family or a badly managed business, never relaxes sufficiently to fully recuperate from stress. Disease then follows close at hand. Any healer who would behave rudely or harshly in public fails to understand health and the interdependence of all people. We are social animals, and to be healthy when surrounded by social disorder or much illness is far more difficult than to be healthy in the opposite sort of surroundings.

On the second level of healing are the behaviors that maintain and comfort chronically ill or limited people. Knowing that little if any recovery is possible from these persons' conditions, kindness and comfort are extended to them. Also on this level is comforting and reassuring people during an acute illness.

On the third level of healing are interventions that aggressively intrude into the patient's body, "assaulting" the symptom. The most extreme example of this is surgery. Any invasion of the body violates the integrity of its system of energy and harms it, although it may also be of benefit. In therapies such as these, the symptom is seen as an enemy who must be fought. This is the most common model of western (allopathic) medicine: the symptom is the enemy and must be obliterated.

Symptoms or illnesses, however unwanted, are not one's enemies; they are the experience of the inefficiency of one's energy flow.

The symptom expresses internal disorder and the need for healing as well as for changing one's ways. All the methods on the third level of healing engage the patient in a warlike process. Although they may be of some benefit, the necessary condition of true healing is love. Third level therapies are not loving by their nature.

Health is unimpeded energy flowing through a person. Ill health is the opposite. Disease is not what it is imagined to be in our culture—a predator that randomly attacks the innocent. Instead, it is the end result of inadequate or deviated energy flow. This causes disease by either undernourishing or deforming specific organs. This is not to deny the existence of bacteria, viruses, parasites, fungi, and so forth; but a person with strong and healthy energy flow will rarely be vulnerable to these.

At the fourth level, healing is cooperative with the nature of the patient. It is only at this level and above that the healer is an ally of the patient's energy during a natural, unforced process of change. It is difficult for westerners with their intellectual and technical approach to problem solving to behave this way in the presence of illness.

Fourth level therapies are not only cooperative with the patient's energy, but can occur only when the patient is in an environment of healthy energy. In these therapies the patient is treated by being near or within a superior system of energy. This system of energy is sometimes a location and sometimes a person. The patient's energy spontaneously imitates the energy of the more highly organized system, resulting in beneficial change. This is why the principal message of this book is to spend time attentively with nature every day. Interestingly, herbalism and apprenticeship to a master also work by this principle. In herbalism the diseased organ of the patient imitates the healthy energy of a selected plant. In apprenticeship, the student imitates the more ideally organized energy of the master. In both, the patient unconsciously imitates energy that is organized in a manner superior to and thus healthier than his or her own.

Levels of Healing

Healing by a loving mediator
using his/her energy skillfully
as an interface between the
patient and nature's energy

Examples

5

-The work of specific healers who may
or may not be associated with various
methods or modalities of healing

-Healing as taught at the Institute of Light

Non-intrusive Therapy

4

-Personally interacting with the energy of nature
-Hands-on healing e.g. Therapeutic Touch™
-Herbalism
-Apprenticeship with a master

Intrusive Therapy

3

-Surgery
-Drug Therapy
-Rolfing™
-Acupuncture
-Reflexology

**Comforting,
Nursing**

2

-Sustaining the sick
-Providing
companionship
-Helping
-Encouraging

**Appropriate and Orderly
Social Behaviors**

1

-Following rules
and laws
-Mannerliness
-Consideration
-Warmth

Other conditions that add to healing by this principle are time spent in natural settings, fresh food and physical exercise outdoors. These obvious prescriptions, although they appeal to common sense, are scarcely subscribed to in this society. Consequently they are not made convenient. To choose what is not considered normal or convenient requires determination. Hence, part of the healer's task, even at this level, is encouraging obvious and simple realities. If these obvious routes to health were acknowledged in our culture, hospitals would be in park-like settings, and physicians would stroll with their patients.

The highest forms of healing, those on the fifth level of the diagram, are those that most improve the organization of one's energy movement. The simpler the pattern of one's flow, the healthier and happier one is. Such an improvement in health is not available from another person, no matter how skilled s/he may be.

At this level of healing, the healer understands fully that s/he is not the source of the healing and that the word healer is a misnomer. S/he does nothing to the patient. Such a healer understands that the highest level of improvement available to people is not from a healer, but through a healer. S/he further understands that true healing can only come from nature's energy. S/he knows that we live immersed in an environment of energy, and that it generally requires the joining together of two people to access its healing or transformative capacity. One of these two is the patient or person in need; the other is the healer who, at the moment of healing, is devoted to serving the needs of the patient. S/he will do the work of mediating between the patient and the environment, functioning like the lens of a camera that brings the light to the film in a way that could not happen without a lens. Even this is not enough. To do this well, the healer must have skillful access to the energy of the Earth and must be in a loving state during this process.

Fine healing also requires that the healer is not personally involved in the outcome. S/he must not take the presence of the symptom or the future progress of the disease personally. S/he assumes responsibility for his or her own preparation and performance as the mediator of the healing, but no responsibility for the outcome. To do so would be utter grandiosity. This is not to say that the healer is indifferent or not hoping for beneficial outcome. Still, s/he realizes that s/he is not the source of the healing, but merely the nexus through which it passes.

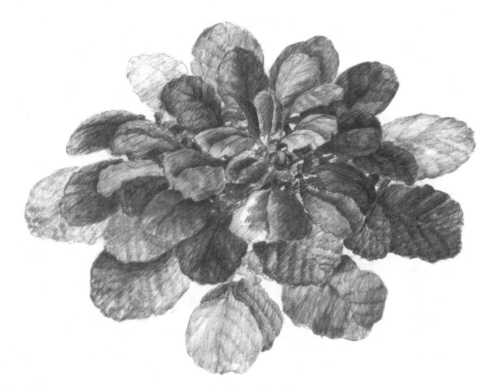

27 Transformation and Work

Ideally, healing improves the organization of much of the energy configuration that is a person. If healing is successful on this scale and the recipient takes advantage of this opportunity to change his or her behavior, s/he is in a sense no longer the same person. S/he is a better person.

Imagine yourself being transformed in this way and becoming superior to how you were previously. You would be wiser and more insightful. You would have more highly developed ethics and values. You would be more energetic and optimistic. You would be kinder and more generous. What would happen then? How might this affect your relationships? What would your job be like if you were to do it more sensitively and ethically? There might be some poorly fitting aspects to your life, once you had improved. It is

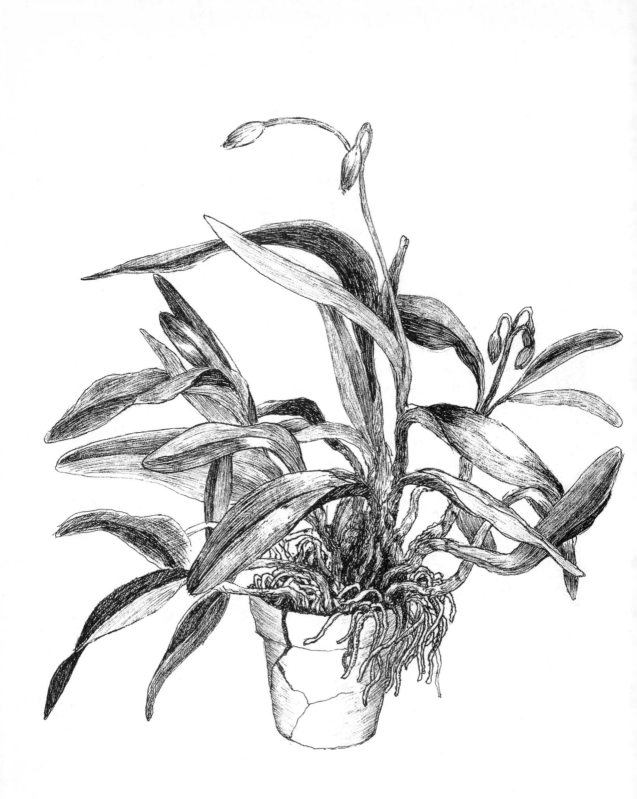

one's career that most easily becomes ill–fitting after substantial healing occurs. Without appropriate work which benefits others, one feels unsatisfied and one's daily work soon degrades into drudgery. Resentment easily follows this. Satisfaction and joy in daily work require that the work itself be meaningful, that it fit the nature of the worker, and that it be done with an open heart. Serving others is not about altruism. It is about satisfaction.

The more efficient one's energy organization is, the more one needs to serve others in order to feel fulfilled.

The more efficient one's energy organization, the greater the goodness one can provide for others.

The greater the goodness one provides, the greater the benefit that all people receive, as our behavior and our energy touches our whole species like ripples expanding through water.

28. Healer as Parent

A mother is the representative of the Earth. Actually, she is the child's connection to the Earth's energy. The Earth's generosity is never contingent upon the worthiness of people's behavior. The Earth feeds us no matter how reprehensible our actions are. A good mother, like the Earth, loves her babies indiscriminately, unconditionally. In teaching someone to live in a healthier way, the healer must sometimes love unconditionally like a mother. This unvarying input of love supports that person to do what s/he previously perceived as frightening, foreign or undesirable. Much healing requires this way of loving, whether from a male or female healer.

Sometimes, however, this is insufficient to promote the other person's best interests, especially if s/he is locked into unhealthy or socially inappropriate behavior, such as drug use, abusive treatment of others or failed responsibilities. The healer, male or female, must then change to a more paternal style of loving—loving combined with demand for appropriate behavior. If a healthy mother is the agent of the Earth, a healthy father is the agent of society, representing the needs of others to the child. When a person's behavior toward others or even toward himself is clearly wrong, the healer does not close his or her heart. S/he opens his or her heart and says simply and clearly, "You must stop," or "You must never do that again."

Most of the demands for good behavior we have heard in our lives were spoken in anger or at least with a closed heart. This evoked a spontaneous defensive response from many of us. Others of us responded with shame or humiliation. This way of demanding change may have been expedient, but it was not healthy in the long run.

With an open heart the healer combines the energies of love with clear limit setting. S/he demands right behavior, but does so

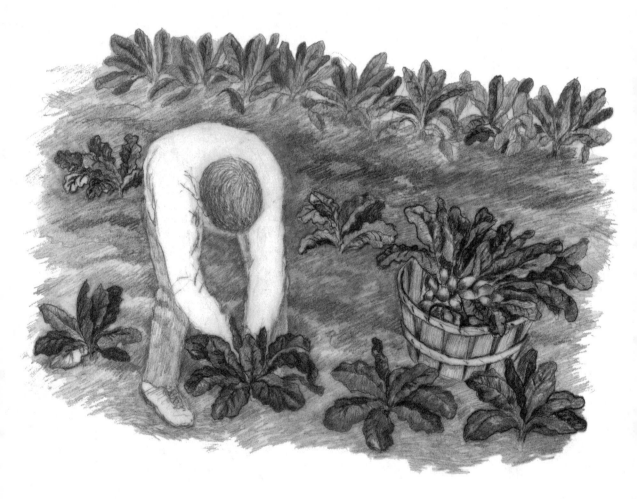

without anger. In the face of this, a person may well change a harmful behavior that has existed for years, as s/he has been presented with the energy key—the demand for right behavior, stated lovingly.

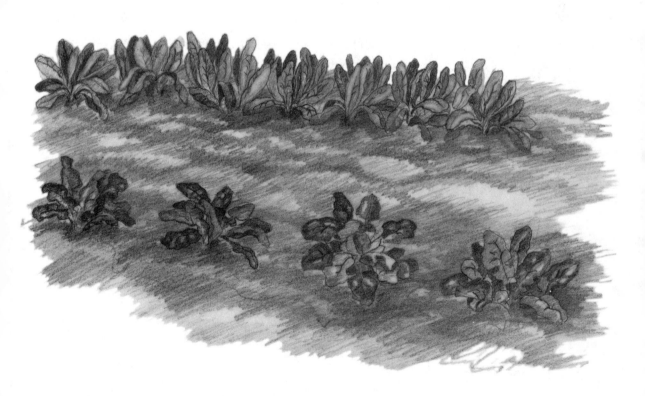

29. Knowing

Theories are attempts to piece together insufficient information into orderly patterns; the goal of a theory is to discover lawfulness and thus predictability in nature.

Theorizing in conventional medicine or psychotherapy, although it may sometimes be helpful, is speculative. Good healers are not speculative, they are descriptive—or at least correlative, describing the concurrence of symptom and energy.

Once a healer is competent, s/he requires precious little theory to guide his or her work. Instead s/he works by paying attention to the patient's problematic energy and then responding to it with his or her love and vigor. The cause of the symptom may be unknown, but the treatment can often proceed successfully without knowing the cause.

Diagram of Healing

Patient
lacks efficient energy flow, which shows itself in physical, psychological and/or spiritual symptoms.

Healer
mediates between nature's energy and the patient by loving and by accessing nature's energy.

Nature's Energy
has the capacity to heal or reorganize the patient's energy flow so it is more efficient.

By what venue does the healer know? S/he knows through two places in his or her intelligence, that is, his or her energy flow: the fourth and sixth chakras (heart and forehead). The sixth chakra is the energy center that can access information which may not be available through the intellect. This is not wisdom. This is information. Is this information certain? Probably not, as every sixth chakra is part of a particular person and its information is delimited by that person's personality and needs. The fourth chakra, the other venue of knowing, has special prejudices. It is a heart and its knowing is colored by love and sympathy. So we must know the limitations of the healer's ways of knowing as well as the limitations of empirical ways of knowing.

Knowing is never absolute, whether it is intuitive or empirical. Ways of knowing vary. Courageous people must accept this and resist the twentieth century mythology that the scientific method is humanity's final triumph in the search for truth.

It is also unnecessary to use occult beliefs, oriental cosmologies, religious dogmas or rituals in order to do healing. One must merely perceive what actually is so. However, clear perception of energy will be difficult if the healer's own energy does not flow optimally, undeterred by physical or emotional illness. Difficulty may also occur if the healer fails to trust his or her own experience of the energy of nature and instead relies on theories or belief systems s/he has learned from others. The healer who wishes to perceive energy without distortion must be healthy, simple in life style and devoid of the motive to use this information selfishly or hurtfully.

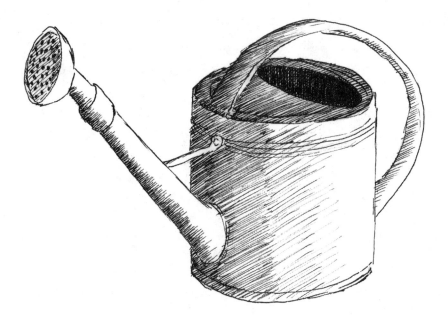

30. Experiencing Nature's Energy

What is nature's energy? Words cannot adequately communicate
this fundamental reality of life. Only experience can do that. If one
does not have experience of the energy of nature, one is left with
nothing other than conventional or theoretical beliefs. These are, at
best, someone else's experience.

A healer is privileged to join with the energy of nature to make
others' lives better. Each time a healer joins in this way with
nature, s/he participates in what may be the ultimate experience.
Each time the healer helps to make life better for one person, s/he
makes life better for those surrounding that person. When a person
is healed and also commits to healthier behavior, the world
literally becomes a better place.

Clearly, a great deal of healing needs to take place in order to make a significant change in our troubled society. It can only be done via nature's energy, a force unknown to many who are lost in the synthetic world of commerce and technology.

The experiencing of nature's energy, interacting with the context that provides us with life, should not only be part of the preparation of all healers; it should also be part of the preparation of physicians, nurses, teachers, parents, managers and any others who want to improve life. Without the experience of nature's energy, one soon becomes uninspired and subsequently loses optimism and commitment to life's work.

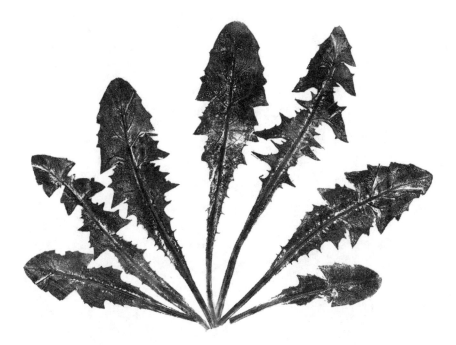

Healing Exercises

Introduction

Learning each of these exercises is like learning a sport. Ideally, it is done with someone who is already skilled. If this is not possible, the next best way is to work with any partner. This way, you will, in a very real sense, pool your energy. Ideally, choose someone who is healthy, has common sense and is peaceful. A female partner would probably be your best choice, given that women generally have more access to the Earth's energy than men.

Keep in mind that the means to make these exercises life changing and even transformative is your attentiveness (see the chapter on attention). Done without concentration, the exercises can be comforting and pleasant, but they will not have the potential healing power that you may hope for.

Never do these exercises under three circumstances: 1) if you do not want to do them; 2) if you are angry; 3) or, if you are using your will or endurance to do the exercises. In all three cases, you will induce the activity of your sympathetic nervous system and eliminate any benefit that comes from these exercises or any other healthy activity.

Keep a journal of your daily experiences. Use words, pictures, diagrams, charts and colors. A record will help you to process new information and more fully understand events in your body and psyche that correlate to doing the exercises.

How long should each exercise be done? Longer is not necessarily better. One guideline is, as long as you can comfortably pay attention. Another is, stop when it is no longer pleasant. Finally (after an initial three weeks), do each one until you feel finished. With experience, you will know when you are done. Your body will feel complete.

Most of the students at the Institute of Light, which is in Cleveland, Ohio where it is cold six months out of the year, do these exercises on plastic drop cloths, exercise mats or sleeping bag mattresses. Don't be afraid that synthetic material will stop the enormous energy of the Earth. There may be some minimal loss, but not nearly the amount of loss that you would have by being wet and/or cold, which will cause you to tighten in discomfort and consequently lose your receptiveness to the Earth's energy. Dress as if it were twenty degrees colder than it is, as you will not be moving. A rain suit and a ski suit are a fine way to make yourself comfortable and free of constraint in what can ironically turn out to be some of the most delightful weather. Although it is best to do these exercises upon arising, if you can't or won't, do them at another time. A less stringent rule would be, do them when you are not tired. If your neighbors want to know why you are doing these things, invite them to join you or explain it as "a healthy meditation, something like yoga."

Almost all of these exercises are to be done outdoors. If one seeks to improve one's own energy, one must go to the source of energy, nature.

If you are ill or in pain these exercises become all the more valuable and important. Ideally do them twice a day. There is a mistaken belief in our society that the sick belong indoors and will worsen if exposed to the elements. This is a complete reversal of the truth. Do not fear going outdoors because you are not feeling well. That is where you can access the energy that will quickly make you healthy again.

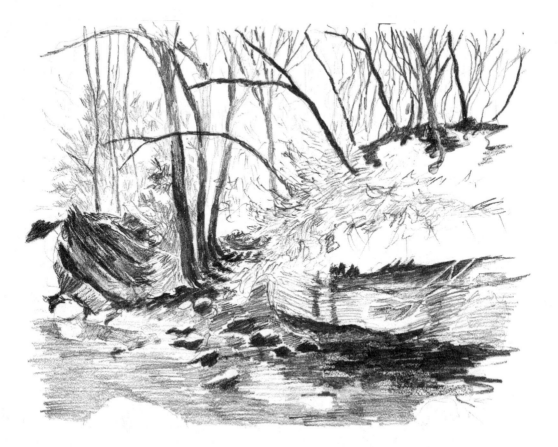

1. Lying down

The first step in approaching the study of energy is to pay attention to the largest and primary source of energy, the Earth. The Earth is an ongoing energy process that feeds, supports and heals us. If you seek health, you must go to the Earth, attentively, every day of your life.

EXERCISE 1. Lie on your back on the Earth. Use a blanket, sleeping bag or a plastic drop cloth if it is cold or wet. Quiet yourself. Pay full attention to the sensations of your spine against the ground. Release the spine; drop it; let it go; relax it into the Earth. This single skill, the releasing of the spine, is the single most tension-reducing behavior. In so doing, one releases a large number of muscles which allows many organs to settle into healthier positions. Most people find this easier to do if they divide the spine into several sections—for example pelvis, lower back, waist, upper back, neck and head—and attend to each section separately.

EXERCISE 2. After a few days of exercise 1, pay attention to the Earth "through" the spine, as if you could see through or reach through your spine into the Earth. As the spine is the central conduit of your life's energy, it easily interacts with the Earth. The length of time of this exercise is determined by the length of your attention span. These exercises will increase your attention span if done daily. Again, it is easier to do this exercise a segment at time.

After a few days of paying attention into the Earth via your released spine, sense farther yet into the Earth, extending your attention down farther into the Earth. Each day you will become more skilled and able to lie attentively a bit longer.

The result of this exercise is to calm yourself as you release "waste" energy into the Earth. At the same time it provides a way of learning about the Earth in a personal and intimate way. Many experience subjectively "entering" the Earth. You will find that this calming, quieting experience is the best way to start and end each day. Try this for one month.

Do not fear the weather when doing this or any of the exercises. Dressing warmly, you can lie on a blanket and/or a plastic drop cloth in the snow or rain and find special benefits that are not available in more temperate weather. Until one has had the experience of lying relaxed in snow or rain, cold or heat, one does not know deeply that nature is safe.

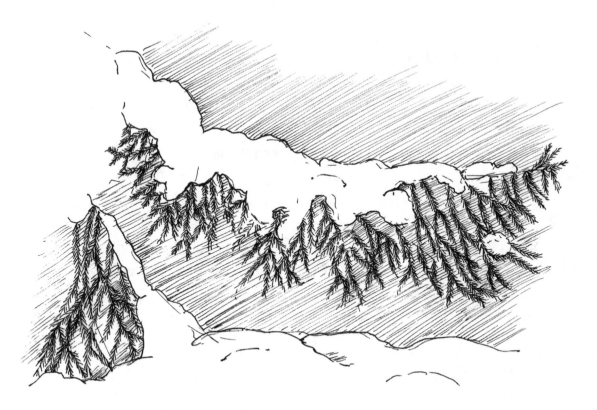

2. Standing

EXERCISE 3. The single most important skill for all who would be healers or who would be healthy, is standing while connecting to the Earth's energy through your feet. Remove your shoes and stand silently on grass or soil. If your feet are too cold, wear shoes or boots; it will still work. This alone, standing barefoot and wordlessly, is a fine beginning. Continue to do this for a minute or two.

Next, stand with all of your attention feeling the sensations of your feet against the Earth. Pay complete attention to the sensations of your feet against the Earth. Each time you lose your concentration, return gently to the task by wiggling your toes. This is how to develop your connection to the Earth. It is done by concentration.

As you practice this each day try giving yourself slightly different directions (only one direction per day), such as: soften the feet, open the feet, drop the feet into the ground, sink into the ground or allow the feet to enter the ground. Some people concentrate better without verbal cues, paying attention only to the sensations of the feet.

EXERCISE 4. A week or two later, increase the level of difficulty. Standing barefoot and silent, aim your attention through the soles of your feet, like beams of light, into the Earth. This version of the exercise, when done with attentiveness and regularity, can be more empowering than any other single energy practice.

By attending downwards through the soles of the feet into the Earth, the body becomes more easily filled with the Earth's energy. A natural and spontaneous process is evoked by attentively joining with the source of life. The length of time needed to master this process is not important. Each person is on their own individual learning "path" and it can not be validly compared with another's.

In the beginning you may have little sensation of filling with energy, but if you practice attentively for a few days you will begin to experience changes. Sensation will probably be felt first in the feet and legs and then in the upper body. This may be felt as tingling, warmth, calmness, fullness, pleasure, relaxation, expansion or vibration. All people are not equally sensitive to this experience. However, their individual level of sensation does not reflect their success. Sensitivity is affected by one's personality, physical structure, diet, and sometimes the presence of drugs in the system.

It will become apparent that this exercise must be done every day, actually a number of times every day—each time that you want to reinstate or increase your flow of energy. This could be upon arising in the morning, when tired after a meal, when in pain, or, certainly, when frightened. Never attempt to heal another person, whether by conventional means or by energy healing methods, without first filling with energy via your feet. Never! To attempt a healing without first instating the flow of the Earth's energy through yourself is to heal not with the Earth's vast supply of energy, but with your own meager resources. This results in personal depletion. If done frequently, it ends in disease.

This practice also can and should be done indoors. During the day you will frequently want more energy and the many changes it brings. Indoor practice will increase your energy. However, only doing it outdoors on the ground has a healing effect.

3. Feet, health and healing

Feet are the principal interface with the Earth's energy, the source of life. Consequently, the method in which we use our feet greatly affects input of energy, release of waste energy and the functioning of the entire body.

The energy flowing through all of the organs and chakras begins and ends at the feet. Because of this, the feet release some of the waste energy emitted from each of these sites.

Something extremely serious went awry in that period when human inventiveness and, worse yet, fashion, began to be valued above our connection to nature. Footgear, at least non-ergonomic footgear, began to interfere with people's connection to the Earth. It also began to interfere with healthy movement.

The foot has a natural walking movement which is seldom experienced while in shoes. Only extensive barefoot walking over irregular surfaces allows this. Although the toes naturally reach and then push off at the end of each step, in our shoe-restrained state most people end each step before this happens.

At present one often cannot go barefoot. Without the resultant free movement, the feet cannot learn their appropriate movement spontaneously and so must be deliberately educated. They must be trained into flexibility, power, vitality and optimal movement. This can be done by various exercises that you can learn from a well-trained dancer; much barefoot walking (with great attentiveness to the sensations of the toes); and massaging the feet daily. Choice of shoes will be self-evident once your feet have begun to move more articulately. Go barefoot as often as you can. Cleanse the waste energy from your feet each day by standing attentively on the Earth (see exercises 3 and 4). Finally, be sure to dance, walk, run, play and/or exercise outdoors every single day. Health is not possible without daily outdoor activity.

After the preparation described above, walk meditatively each day paying attention to the sensations of the toes. This is easiest to feel while walking uphill.

A result of this training regime is significant correction of the way your legs and torso muscles move as you walk. The torso's internal muscles, principally the ileo-psoas, become activated by increased use of the toes (examine these muscles in an anatomy diagram; see how they form a principal source of internal power and movement for the human body).

We exist by way of three possible connections from the Earth to the first chakra: seat, knees or feet. The feet are thus organs of access to the essence; through your feet you participate in the power and health of nature's energy.

4. Standing with a tree

Now that you have developed some skill at standing and joining with the Earth, it is time to go further and study with a master of this art, a tree.

Trees are the great masters of accessing the Earth's energy and allowing it to flow upwards through their physical structures. Although the tree is a different life form from yourself, it still qualifies as a master with whom to study, as all organisms share nature's energy. Although any tree is a master of linear flow, some are more powerful than others. Find a tall, straight deciduous tree (one that looses its leaves in autumn) with which to stand.

EXERCISE 5. Stand silently facing a tree. Approach to within an arm's length and begin exercise number four, the standing exercise. Step back. Stroll about, paying attention to the sensations in your body and to your emotional state.

EXERCISE 6. A few minutes later, try the entire exercise with your back to the tree. It is not necessary to lean on or touch the tree, as its energy extends well past its physical structure (as does yours). Make entries in your journal describing and comparing the two forms of this exercise.

In your next encounter with a tree, repeat either version of the exercise. Then stand there and maintain your silence for as long as possible. It will be easier to be silent in the tree's presence than by yourself.

On another day, repeat this exercise in a seated position. Compare this with the standing version. Do not do your standing exercises with trees all the time. Their energy is much larger than yours and you do not want to become dependent on this extra energy support for your success.

5. Standing on different surfaces

EXERCISE 7. Begin by doing the standing exercise indoors and then repeat it outdoors. Compare these. Then, find a variety of soils and natural surfaces on which to do the standing exercise, comparing your experiences on each of them. Some possibilities are rock, clay, topsoil, humus and sand. Attending to the differences in standing on various materials will refine your perception of energy. It will also reveal a variety of resources, as each form of Earth offers you a somewhat different gift. Once you can feel the differences, try doing your standing work in a variety of locations such as forests, swamps, fields, hills, valleys and so forth, comparing these experiences.

Find a favorite surface on which to stand. What is it that you prefer about this?

EXERCISE 8. After doing the standing exercise, take a handful of your favorite form of earth and hold it against the center of your chest. Focus your attention at the place where your chest and the Earth meet. Silently keep your attention at the meeting point for a few minutes. What did you feel in your chest? How were your emotions affected? What happened to your energy state in general? Under what circumstances would you want to repeat it? What could be healed in this way?

For a week, begin each day doing the standing exercise on your favorite substance. Follow this with a meditation holding this substance against your heart. How does this prepare you for the day?

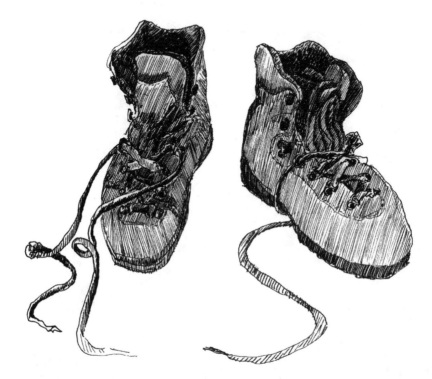

6. Cleansing

Cleansing is ridding yourself of energy whose frequency does not match your own inherent energy.

Each person is a composite of several frequencies of energy. Other frequencies, although possibly healthy for another person may be unhealthy for you. The unwanted energy reduces efficiency and can cause illness. There are also very low frequencies of energy that are unhealthy for any person. These seem to be the result of negative emotions, drugs, unhealthy food and environmental pollutants.

It is important to learn to cleanse your energy every day in order to stay healthy and efficient. Here are two ways to cleanse your energy:

EXERCISE 9. Lie on the ground and cleanse one chakra at a time by paying attention to the back of that chakra (that place on your spine) where it meets the ground (refer to the chakra chart). Do this until you feel, see or sense a change. Ignore the seventh chakra (on top of your head); functioning like a chimney, it usually cleans itself.

EXERCISE 10. Stand with your back against a tree and do the same.

For best results, precede and follow cleansing by doing the standing exercise.

Begin exercises nine and ten by cleansing the sixth chakra, as it regulates the rest of the system and will do so more efficiently while you continue the cleansing. After this, work sequentially from the first chakra upwards.

You could cleanse only a single chakra if that is all that is of concern to you. For example, if your eyes burn, you might pause and cleanse the sixth chakra.

Exercise, especially vigorous exercise, helps the cleansing process: it causes the movements of the chakras (they are always in motion) to increase. If you have reason to believe that you are in need of considerable cleaning, follow the above procedures with dancing or running.

Always cleanse yourself after participating in a healing. No matter how good your energy usage skills may be, it is possible that your energy was vulnerable in some way to the waste energy released by the other person.

It is also helpful to keep candles burning or a fire in the fireplace in whatever place you do healing. This will burn off most types of waste energy. Better yet, do healing outdoors and you can leave the cleanup work for the Earth.

Never leave uncovered beverages in the place you do healing, as fluids "attract" waste energy.

7. Standing in the winter

Many people dread the cold. If you do these exercises every day, no matter what the weather, you will begin to feel at home on the Earth all the time. This is important, as fear, in this case fear of cold weather, prevents calm feelings which are a necessary precondition for health.

EXERCISE 11. When the weather becomes cold and the Earth begins to harden, go outdoors and remove your shoes and socks. Stand quietly. Aim directly down through your feet (the standing exercise). How do your feet feel? What is the effect of energy flow on body temperature? What hypothesis do you now have about staying warm in cold weather?

Do this exercise barefoot each day until the first snow fall. If you have had some success, try it in the snow. Bear in mind that some cultures conduct their daily lives in the snow. If you are uncomfortable, do your standing work during the winter with footgear, as more energy is lost by tightening against cold than by grounding yourself through galoshes.

8. Sitting on the Earth

Whether standing or sitting, accessing the Earth's energy is done in the same way. One must aim or reach downwards into the Earth. This induces energy flow, which then follows the length of the spine upwards to and even past the top of the head. When standing you reach downwards from the feet. When sitting you reach downwards from the seat.

EXERCISE 12. Find a place to sit on the ground, dressing so that your clothing doesn't bind. Sitting erectly but not rigidly, pay attention to your seat against the Earth. For many, sitting cross-legged is difficult. If you cannot do this or cannot do this without slouching, support your back by leaning against something, possibly a tree. Another means to accomplish this is to raise the buttocks by sitting on a rolled blanket or a dense cushion. With closed eyes, search for the place that is obviously the center of the seat. This is not a logical search for the center. Pay attention and the center will become apparent. After you know where the center is, reach beneath you and touch the center. What anatomical structure is this? Repeat the exercise and see if you produce the same or different results. Why should this place be the center?

EXERCISE 13. Sit on the Earth quietly and focus all your attention at the center of your seat. Do this for several minutes. Describe what happens.

Attending to the center of your seat, the bottom of the spine's energy, is very much like attending to the soles of the feet. By focusing your attention, you induce spontaneous energy flow from the Earth, just as you do when standing and attending to your feet.

EXERCISE 14. The next day, sitting on the Earth, attend to the center of your seat and aim down through the center of your seat into the Earth. Continue until your body is flowing with energy. Proceed as if you were standing.

Do this daily for a week. Do this sitting cross-legged on the Earth or floor, as well as in chairs. Many people can not sit in a cross-legged position at all. If you are one of them, do your seated work in a chair. Compare this exercise with the standing exercise. How are they different? How are they similar? When would you want to do one or the other?

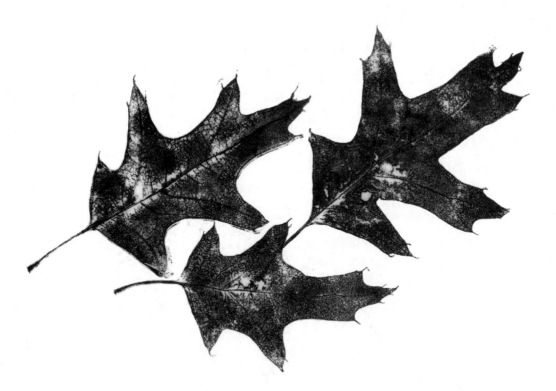

9. Walking

When you have learned to reach into the Earth and to increase your own flow of energy, you are literally ready to move on. Before starting exercise seventeen, examine an anatomical diagram of the perineum. Look at another diagram illustrating the spine and pelvis. Try to understand how they fit together. This will help you to visualize the first chakra emerging from the very bottom of the spine (the coccyx) and then passing through the perineum, which is on the floor of the pelvis.

EXERCISE 15. Begin in the usual way by doing the standing exercise. Momentarily contract the muscles that stop urination. Release them and walk while attending to the resultant lingering sensation. Repeat the momentary muscle contraction each time you loose your concentration.

When you are able to do this exercise for five minutes, try the next one. Begin with the standing exercise. When it is completed, pay attention to the sensations of your spine from waist to neck. Then walk with your attention in that part of the spine that goes from waist to neck, experiencing its sensations (energy flow). When you can walk in this manner for two minutes, proceed to exercise 16.

EXERCISE 16. Begin with the standing exercise, then pay attention to the energy flowing upward along the front of the torso. You will experience it as a delicate sensation lifting your torso. Then walk while attending to that stream of energy. Do this daily for a week.

EXERCISE 17. In the next week, as you walk, alternate paying attention to the spine with paying attention to the front of your torso at approximately two minute intervals. In the following week, if you are able to, integrate them by walking while attending to both your front and your back simultaneously. You will experience being lifted by the flow of your energy. Again, do the standing exercise before this exercise or any significant exertion, in order to have enough energy to help you succeed.

When you are able to do this last exercise you will be able to walk in quiet, efficient comfort. Do it for more extended periods of time. Soon you may be able to do it while walking with others.

Should you feel tired while walking, never forget to pause and do the standing exercise. By reinstating your energy connection with the Earth, you will increase your power. This is also the way to quickly get past a moment of fear, small or large.

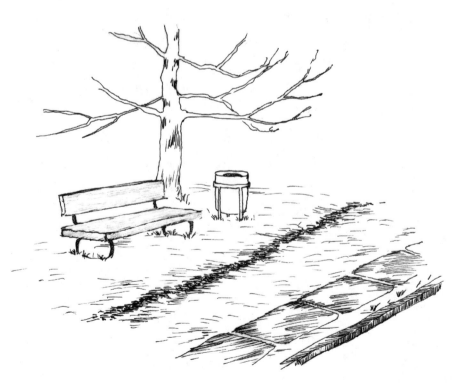

10. Sitting in silence

You have learned to stand and walk more skillfully. Now you must use your improved concentration and energy usage to do a more traditional meditation. The goal of this meditation is to sit in silent energy flow. Mastery of this exercise will bring more tranquility to your daily life.

EXERCISE 18. Begin by doing the standing exercise. Then sit in a chair that allows you to keep your back erect, knees a bit apart and feet flat on the floor. If your back is not erect, "walk" your buttocks all the way back into the chair. Proper placement of the buttocks in a chair automatically aligns the spine, if the chair is no deeper than the length of your upper legs. If the chair is deeper, place a cushion behind your back. If your feet do not rest flat on the floor, place a pillow or a phone book beneath them. Gently rest your hands in your lap. Begin by tightening the muscles of urination momentarily. Then, pay attention to the resultant lingering sensation for a minute or two. This generates energy, just as the standing exercise does. When that attending is finished place one or both hands on the center of your chest. Sit with your attention where your hands touch your body, until it becomes difficult. Do not attempt to endure. This exercise is to teach you to sit gently with your attention at your heart, not to engage you in struggle. Always remember to begin with the standing exercise. Repeat this as often as you wish, until you can do this with comfort for about two minutes. Then move on to the next exercise.

EXERCISE 19. Prepare by doing the standing exercise. Next, sit in the prescribed manner (see exercise 18). Place your hands and your attention on your chest. Sit silently in this manner. Now proceed with any activity that is best prepared for by calmness, such as eating, resting, meeting with a colleague, or beginning your day. Use preparing for action with calmness as frequently as you wish.

Once you become more skilled at this exercise, do it while listening to someone speak. At first this will be difficult; but soon you will find this not only possible, but a way to provide calmness and support for yourself as well as the other person.

This meditation is made possible by all of your prior work. It is your energy flow that supports your attention. Without the preparatory step of increasing your energy flow, meditation can only be an exercise of will or self–restraint. Doing it that way easily causes frustration or guilt.

Meditation is not esoteric or arcane. It is a daily activity to keep you healthy and calm. It improves your health and prepares you for healing others.

11. Eating

Now you are ready to eat peacefully. If you do, it will substantially improve your health and the quality of your daily life. It may not have been previously possible to do this, as you did not have the energy skills to allow calm eating.

EXERCISE 20. Begin by doing the standing exercise. Then, sit alone at the table as if you were sitting to meditate. Pay attention to the center of your chest. Then, without reading or talking, without music or television, take one bite of food. When you are done with that first bite, lay down your fork. Pause and pay attention to the center of your chest. Then begin the next bite of food.

At first, do not eat an entire meal in this new way. Eat half of it as described above and half in the old way. Compare the two halves. For a week, begin all meals this way. How long do you last before lapsing into habit?

In the next week, try to eat a complete meal this way. Eat this meal alone and in silence. Pause as often as you need. How does this affect your appetite and your mood? If you suffer from high cholesterol or high blood pressure, have your condition evaluated after two weeks of eating in this way. If you are overweight, pay attention to the scale at the beginning and end of two weeks of this practice.

Meditative eating puts the digestive organs into an ideal (parasympathetic) state in which to do their work. Their efficiency is increased and less energy is needed for digestion. This leaves more energy available for your other activities. If you suffer from any chronic problems with digestion or elimination, this practice may be revelatory.

12. Resting

It is time to rest when concentration has diminished, the body feels uncomfortable, and the emotions are more difficult to manage. Most of us are on a three hour cycle; every three hours we must rest briefly.

EXERCISE 21. Lie on your back. Place your left hand on the center of your chest and the right hand on your hip. Wordlessly, pay attention to the sensation of your hand against your chest. Do so until there is a shift in your feelings. The shift will feel like being smoothed or eased. Do not rest any longer than that or you will begin to lose energy.

When you are done with this structured rest, rise and do the standing exercise. This "re-starts" your energy flow. It is possible to rest sitting up, but it is a bit more difficult. Try it both ways and compare them.

You have learned to use energy to support your basic activities: standing, sitting, walking, eating and resting. If you do these activities quietly and mindfully your life will be transformed into an easier one.

It is the daily integration of good energy practice into your ordinary life that will make you into a healthy person and a fine healer. Being a healer is not something that is done in isolated moments called healing sessions; it is how you live and how that in turn affects others.

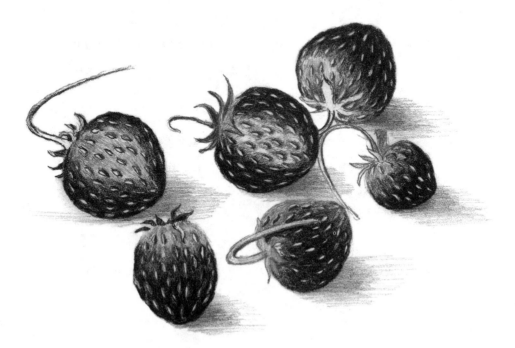

13. Attending to the heart

Begin by doing exercise 18.

After a few days of doing exercise number 18 you will become aware of a sensation of expansion in your chest. For the next few days, begin the exercise and then pay attention to the subtle expansion of the chest, but do not try to expand it willfully. Allow it to expand and pay attention to that. After each meditation, stroll around paying attention to your physical and emotional state. Try to describe what you feel in words.

You are beginning to practice love, but that is little more than sentiment unless it is done with sufficient power. The standing or sitting exercise is not mere preparation, but accessing the power of the Earth to turn your love into love that has enough power to improve your life and the lives of those about you.

EXERCISE 22. In the second week do the standing exercise and then sit while wordlessly paying attention to the center of your chest. This time, take your attention an inch or two into your chest (towards the spine) and hold it there for a minute or two. Do this exercise at least twice daily for a week.

You are entering your fourth chakra. As you continue to do this you will find that it induces feelings of happiness, love and calm. You may do this as frequently as you like. The more often you do this the better your life will become. Do not try to do it if you are angry, frightened or tired.

In our first set of exercises, you focused on your longitudinal energy flow, accessing energy support from the Earth. Now you are beginning to expand or widen your energy. These practices are not done instead of longitudinal flow; they are done in addition to it. They are the second step.

If you were never to go farther in your work, but were to practice all the prior teachings and paying attention to the heart, your life would be substantially improved.

14. Using your heart in other situations

Now it is time to sit with an open heart in the presence of another person. It is far more pleasant and effective than the more conventional way of being with people. Begin with simple tasks.

EXERCISE 23. Sit with others in the family while in this state, but not while watching television or listening to loud music. Sit with your attention in your heart (in the center of your chest) and watch a child.

EXERCISE 24. Pay attention to your heart while you are with the checkout person in the grocery store. Do this with the bank teller and a clerk in a retail shop. Do this before speaking on the telephone. The list, of course is limitless. As you begin to conduct interactions with your heart open, you are becoming a true healer.

In Conclusion

These exercises teach the core abilities whose mastery will make you into a person of health and goodness.

The practices with nature use natural energy configurations to teach and improve you. They are the needed daily reminders of who you really are—part of the Earth, part of nature.

To be a healer is to be master of your own energy flow. If you do this, those who are in your presence will unconsciously imitate the superior level of your energy organization and find themselves improved.